P9-DDD-340

"I recommend this groundbreaking book to all my clients."

—Diane Wiessinger, MS, IBCLC

"I fell in love with this book; every page is a jewel. It simply 'delivers' what every mother needs—the natural laws to build a breastfeeding relationship. Understanding the first forty days has changed the way I talk to new parents and teach breastfeeding supporters. Finally, here is a book that talks about breastfeeding without all the rules. This book lives in my bag to share with everyone!"

—Carrie Finger, BFA, IBCLC, LCCE, lactation program director at Aviva Institute

Breastfeeding Made Simple

SEVEN NATURAL LAWS
for NURSING MOTHERS

SECOND EDITION

NANCY MOHRBACHER, IBCLC, FILCA
KATHLEEN KENDALL-TACKETT, PH.D., IBCLC

New Harbinger Publications, Inc.

Publisher's Note

This publication is designed to provide accurate and authoritative information in regard to the subject matter covered. It is sold with the understanding that the publisher is not engaged in rendering psychological, financial, legal, or other professional services. If expert assistance or counseling is needed, the services of a competent professional should be sought.

NEW HARBINGER PUBLICATIONS is a registered trademark of New Harbinger Publications, Inc.

Distributed in Canada by Raincoast Books

Copyright © 2010 by Nancy Mohrbacher and Kathleen Kendall-Tackett
New Harbinger Publications, Inc.
5674 Shattuck Avenue
Oakland, CA 94609
www.newharbinger.com

All Rights Reserved

Acquired by Tesilya Hanauer; Cover design by Amy Shoup; Edited by Elisabeth Beller

Library of Congress Cataloging-in-Publication Data

Mohrbacher, Nancy.
  Breastfeeding made simple : seven natural laws for nursing mothers / Nancy Mohrbacher and Kathleen Kendall-Tackett ; foreword by Jack Newman. -- 2nd ed.
    p. cm.
  Includes bibliographical references and index.
  ISBN 978-1-57224-861-8 (pbk.) -- ISBN 978-1-57224-862-5 (pdf ebook)
  1. Breastfeeding. I. Kendall-Tackett, Kathleen A. II. Title.
  RJ216.M5697 2010
  649'.33--dc22

                              2010034325

Printed in the United States of America

23 22 21

25 24 23 22 21 20 19 18

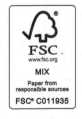

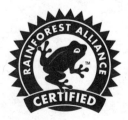

Contents

- Breastfeeding: The Biological Norm for Mothers and Babies
- How to Use This Book

PART I
The Laws

Law 1: *Babies and Mothers Are Hardwired to Breastfeed*

- Your Baby's Hardwiring ◆ Are Mothers Hardwired, Too?
- When the System Breaks Down ◆ Summary

PART II

Applying the Laws

Foreword

How did breastfeeding become so unnecessarily complicated? As the years go by, I am often astounded by how we manage to add new wrinkles of complexity to something that should be easy, natural, and uncomplicated. Of course, breastfeeding itself has not become more complex than it was, say, two hundred years ago. Rather, it is the way we think about breastfeeding that has changed.

As a pediatrician working in southern Africa in the early 1980s, I was amazed at how naturally mothers breastfed their babies. They just put the baby to the breast, with no fuss or bother, no diagrams of how the baby should latch on, no concern about how many minutes the baby nursed on each side, no obsession with how many hours between feedings, no anxiety that the baby had fed only six times a day or fourteen times a day instead of the standard North American eight to twelve times; and no one thought that breastfeeding might not work. And again, to my amazement, it almost always did work.

The very fact that I was amazed, of course, speaks volumes about what I, brought up and trained as a pediatrician in North America, experienced in my life and professional training. These African mothers, the vast majority of whom had never read a book on breastfeeding, who never attended a prenatal class, who probably couldn't imagine what a lactation consultant would do, seemed to exhibit no more anxiety about how they were breastfeeding than about how they were breathing. Of course, breastfeeding was not always problem free in southern Africa either (just as breathing is not always problem free, if you have asthma, for example), but mothers lived in a culture where breastfeeding was normal, and if mothers did run into problems, they had women all around them (their own mothers, sisters, friends) who had breastfed and who usually knew how to get them through it. In fact, the mothers who seemed to have the most problems were those who were the best educated (in the modern sense) and the most Westernized.

However, this basic, ingrained knowledge of how to breastfeed and care for babies was being lost even in southern Africa by the 1980s, when I was there. More and more mothers were having difficulty with "not enough milk," something that older physicians told me they had never heard of. More were using formula supplements, when their own mothers apparently hadn't needed them years before. Part of the problem was the increasing availability of formula and the allure that formula has for poor people ("I can afford to give my baby formula"), even if they couldn't afford it. An equally important part was the greater availability of Western medicine.

Now, Western medicine has accomplished some pretty marvelous things. Our ability to save the lives of babies born as early as twenty-five weeks or even earlier is nothing less than miraculous and was unheard of even fifty years ago (though the long-term results may not always be as wonderful as we would like). Our ability to treat many kinds of cancer that were previously almost always fatal is another. One thing that Western medicine has not done, however, is produce artificial milk that is the same as human milk. Despite marketing strategies to convince us otherwise, what are commonly called formulas are actually very different from mother's milk.

What happened? Why did women in North America and other affluent areas of the world abandon breastfeeding? By the early 1970s only about a quarter of all mothers in North America even started out breastfeeding, and most of them stopped within a few weeks. There were many reasons for this, including the fact that women were returning to outside work shortly after giving birth, as maternity leave was and is virtually nonexistent in the United States. But equally if not more important was that Western medicine had decided that what human beings made in a factory was better than what had served humanity well for hundreds of thousands of generations. (Many more women are now breastfeeding in the United States even though maternity leave is still very short, demonstrating that it is not just outside work that determines breastfeeding rates). How many mothers have come to our breastfeeding clinic, accompanied by their own mothers who told me, "I wanted to breastfeed, but the doctor told me that formula was better"? And this, in the 1960s and 1970s, when formulas weren't as good as they are now (and they're still not up to scratch today and won't be in 2020, either).

When formulas first started to become popular, in the early part of the twentieth century, they were very complicated to make up. Indeed, they were called "formulas" because you took one part of this, another part of that, yet another part of something else, and you had to be very careful to mix the quantities according to the age and size of the baby and their reaction to this milk, which was different than the human milk babies' bodies are designed to eat. Furthermore, the immune-deficient, artificially fed baby had to be protected from foreign bacteria, so complicated instructions on how to sterilize the formula and the bottles and the teats were needed. Physicians often worked hand in hand with the formula manufacturers to encourage formula use because they suddenly had a new reason for patients to come in. Nursing mothers would never have gone, in those days, to see a physician (almost always a man) to ask about breastfeeding issues. They would ask their mothers or sisters. But here was a whole new set of patients, new mothers, who needed to see a doctor to find out how to feed their babies. And with that came information about how to take care of their babies. Rules were needed—otherwise, why would the mother need the doctor? So rules were invented, not only for how to make up formula but also for how often and how long to feed the baby. There were also new rules for child care, rules such as leaving a baby to cry and thus avoiding "spoiling" them by picking them up.

As the years went on, formula preparation became less complicated, with ready-made versions or those that simply needed water added. At the same time, breastfeeding, which had been easy and carefree, became more and more complicated. The rules devised to use in formula preparation and feeding got applied to breastfeeding. After all, when you apply "scientific principles" to feeding an infant with formula, it makes sense that breastfeeding should work exactly as formula feeding does. A brief discussion of just a couple of these many rules will illustrate what I mean.

Feed Every Three to Four Hours

What is it that determines how long a baby should wait between feedings? That's easy—it's the amount of milk they drink. With a bottle, you can force the baby to take more than they really want. If the doctor says the baby should take four ounces, the mother, wishing to obey instructions, tries to make the baby take four ounces, even if the baby really wants only three. This overstuffed child may then sleep three to four hours. With breastfeeding, babies rarely take more than they want, and it's impossible to force them to take more. Not only that, with the poor teaching mothers still receive on how breastfeeding works, babies often get less than they'd prefer, even if the milk supply is abundant. If babies takes only two ounces from the breast, they'll likely wake up in two hours instead of three or four, leading many mothers to these conclusions:

- I don't have enough milk.

- Human milk is not as good as formula.

- Breastfeeding imposes too many demands on me.

Feed for Ten to Twenty Minutes

It takes the average baby about ten to twenty minutes to empty a bottle. Since one bottle is supposed to equal two breasts, the logic says to breastfeed for ten to twenty minutes. It seems to make sense, but when you know the differences between the two systems, the analogy is obviously wrong. The breast does not work at all in the same way as the bottle. The bottle gives steady flow throughout the feeding. But the breast gives less flow until the milk release, then more rapid flow than the bottle, and then it slows down again. A mother may have several milk releases during a feeding, so that flow from breast to baby is often up and down. Suggesting that the baby will get 90 percent of the milk in the first ten minutes, as many physicians still do, assumes the breast is like the bottle—but it's not. If the mother believes the ten-to-twenty-minute rule and the baby takes more than this amount of time to feed, the mother may conclude and may be supported by her doctor in the following:

- ◆ I don't have enough milk.

- ◆ Human milk is not as good as formula.

- ◆ Breastfeeding imposes too many demands on me.

On the other hand, some babies whose mothers have a lot of milk may only feed on one breast for ten or fifteen minutes, or even less, and be perfectly satisfied. But since it takes two breasts to equal one bottle, the mother (and the physician) may conclude that the baby is not getting enough milk.

The Baby Is Not Getting Enough Milk

Applying rules that may or may not be appropriate for artificial feeding is obviously not appropriate for breastfeeding. By trying to squeeze a round peg into a square hole, we have twisted and turned our notions of how to breastfeed so that we've lost sight of what breastfeeding is supposed to be like. And mothers are completely stymied by all the conflicting advice they hear, as each health provider gives them a story that best fits with that health provider's notion of how to fit breastfeeding into that square hole. The most consistent thing I hear from mothers coming to our breastfeeding clinic is that "Every nurse and doctor told me something different."

The truth of the matter is that many health professionals have an intrinsic mistrust of nature. We are taught as pediatricians, for example, that a baby is sick unless proved otherwise. This isn't usually said in so many words, but it is the message behind what we do. The fear of litigation plays a large part in this. As pediatricians, we're always assuming the worst, and when you assume the worst, you find easy ways of avoiding it. So, for example, it is obvious that the exclusively breastfed one-day-old baby is getting much less milk than the artificially fed baby. In a bottlefeeding mentality, it is assumed that there is not enough milk in the first few days, before the "milk comes in." But this is taking the bottlefed baby getting artificial milk as the norm. In fact, artificially fed babies are getting too much in the first few days, and this is not necessarily a good thing.

Breastfeeding Made Simple is exactly what the nursing mother needs these days. Learning the natural laws of breastfeeding will help mothers cut through the nonsense that they may hear about breastfeeding from friends, relatives, the media, and, unfortunately, from their health care providers. By simplifying breastfeeding, it will work better. By simplifying breastfeeding, mothers and babies will be happier. By simplifying breastfeeding, more mothers will breastfeed more exclusively and longer. This is a book that has long been needed.

—Jack Newman, MD, FRCPC
Toronto, Ontario

Introduction

Congratulations! You are about to take part in one of life's great miracles—breastfeeding your baby. For the vast majority of women, breastfeeding is entirely possible. But sometimes women have a hard time. The good news is that breastfeeding can be simple, especially if you know the tricks. And we're here to share them with you.

Allow us to introduce ourselves. We are Nancy and Kathy, and between us, we have more than fifty years of experience working with breastfeeding mothers.

Nancy breastfed her own three sons, Carl, Peter, and Ben, who are now grown, and she has been working with breastfeeding families since 1982. As a board-certified lactation consultant since 1991, Nancy founded and ran a large lactation private practice in the Chicago area for ten years. She is the author of *Breastfeeding Answers Made Simple: A Guide for Helping Mothers* (2010), a book for lactation professionals, and also the coauthor of the popular *Breastfeeding Answer Book* (2003), a research-based counseling guide used by health professionals internationally. In 2008 the International Lactation Consultant Association (ILCA) officially recognized Nancy's lifetime achievements in the field of breastfeeding—as one of the first group of sixteen—by awarding her the designation FILCA, which stands for Fellow of the International Lactation Consultant Association. Nancy now works as a lactation consultant at Ameda Breastfeeding Products, manufacturer of the Ameda breast pumps, where she talks daily to breastfeeding mothers by phone and provides breastfeeding education to health professionals. She also leads a monthly breastfeeding group for families in the Chicago area. She lectures to health care providers around the world.

Kathy breastfed her two sons, Ken and Chris, and is a health psychologist, board-certified lactation consultant, and La Leche League leader. She has been working with breastfeeding families since 1994 and is the former chair of the New Hampshire Breastfeeding Task Force. She now lives in the Texas Panhandle, where she is a clinical associate professor of pediatrics at Texas Tech University School of Medicine in Amarillo and, among her other responsibilities, really enjoys teaching pediatric residents about breastfeeding. She also works with mothers by phone and online, particularly around mental health issues and breastfeeding. Kathy is a Fellow of the American Psychological Association in both health and trauma psychology. She also works as an acquisitions and development editor for Hale Publishing, developing a series of books for both mothers and professionals on breastfeeding.

Kathy's research focuses on the mind-body connection in health, and encompasses such broad-ranging topics as trauma and health, depression in new mothers, and breastfeeding. She has authored or edited twenty books, and authored more than 250 articles, book chapters, and other pieces of work on a wide range of topics in women's health. Some of her most recent books include *Depression in New Mothers*, 2nd ed. (Routledge, 2010); *Non-pharmacologic Treatments for Depression in New Mothers* (Hale Publishing, 2008); and *The Psychoneuroimmunology of Chronic Disease* (American Psychological Association, 2009). Kathy is currently analyzing data from her Survey of Mothers' Sleep and Fatigue—an international study of sleep in mothers of infants. She speaks to audiences of health care providers on these issues around the world.

In this book, we will share with you the simple dynamics—or "natural laws"—of breastfeeding that all good lactation consultants use to help mothers. If you read this book during pregnancy, you can use these natural laws to avoid breastfeeding problems. If you read this book after your baby's birth, you can use these laws to make breastfeeding easier, solve problems, and help meet your breastfeeding goals.

These natural laws are the "secrets" nobody told you about breastfeeding. After generations of bottlefeeding, we are now relearning what women used to know about nursing their babies. If you never had the opportunity to see women breastfeed while you were growing up, learning these natural laws is a must. In a world of conflicting information, you can use them to distinguish good breastfeeding advice from bad.

Breastfeeding: The Biological Norm for Mothers and Babies

As we wrote the first edition of this book, a national advertising campaign promoting breastfeeding was launched in the United States. The primary focus of the Ad Council (the company that made the ads) was to promote exclusive breastfeeding for six months. The slogan of the Ad Council's breastfeeding campaign is "Babies were born to be breastfed," meaning that breastfeeding is the biological norm for mothers and babies. Let's take a look at why the Ad Council chose breastfeeding as an important public-health initiative.

Health Outcomes and Human Milk

In 2009, an article in the April issue of the *Atlantic* described "The Case Against Breastfeeding" (Rosin 2009). And it made headlines around the world. The author, Hanna Rosin, contended that the public had been deceived to believe that mother's milk made huge differences in health—and that it simply wasn't true. In fact, she claimed that breastfeeding was just another way to subjugate women. And why do it at all if it was just going to cause you a lot of stress?

We must respectfully disagree.

At this point, the research studies comparing breastfeeding with man-made substitutes number in the thousands, and the findings show striking differences. Don't take our word for it. We invite you to examine the evidence for yourself and have made some of the major research reviews available on our website (www.breastfeedingmadesimple.com). Researchers have found that during the first year of life, babies fed nonhuman milks have a higher incidence of these health problems:

- respiratory disease, including pneumonia and bronchitis

- diarrhea and other digestive illnesses

- ear infections (up to four times more than babies fed human milk)

- urinary tract infections

- meningitis

- sudden infant death syndrome (SIDS) (Ip et al. 2009)

Babies deprived of human milk's living antibodies are sick more often, have more severe illnesses, and are hospitalized more often and for a longer time (Cunningham, Jelliffe, and Jelliffe 1991). Examining the research worldwide, a 2003 article in the *Lancet* concluded that exclusive breastfeeding for six months by 90 percent of mothers could prevent 13 percent of child deaths—or save 1.3 million children annually (Jones et al. 2003). These findings are not confined to the developing world. A 2004 article in *Pediatrics* reported that 21 percent of U.S. infant deaths between one month and one year of age could be prevented if all U.S. babies did any amount of breastfeeding (Chen and Rogan 2004). Stated another way, what this really means is that infant formula increases U.S. infant deaths during the first year of life by 27 percent. Even more striking, during a baby's first three months, this paper found that exclusive formula feeding increases infant mortality by 61 percent. A 2010 article estimated that each year, exclusive breastfeeding for six months by 90 percent of U.S. mothers could prevent 911 infant deaths and save the U.S. health care system US$13 billion (Bartick and Reinhold 2010).

But the negative health outcomes associated with nonhuman milks are not limited to infancy. Adults who were formula fed as infants have a higher incidence of these health problems:

- allergy

- asthma

- Crohn's disease and other inflammatory bowel diseases

- diabetes (both type 1 and type 2)

- Hodgkin's disease

- childhood leukemia

- celiac disease

- childhood cancers

- breast cancer

- obesity (AAP 2005b; Ip et al. 2007)

The list of health problems associated with formula use continues to grow. In fact, the more we learn, the clearer it becomes that for a baby's immune system to be fully activated after birth, human milk's living antibodies are needed for at least the first twelve months of life.

More Than Food

Your milk is good food for your baby, of course, but it is so much more. At birth, your baby's body expects to receive the unique living components that are in your milk. If your baby is fed nonhuman milks, he will be missing many ingredients essential for normal body function. There are many ways these essential elements affect your baby. But for now we'll take a close look at the impact of human milk on just three aspects of your baby's body: immune function, digestion, and brain development.

NORMAL IMMUNE FUNCTION

Let's begin with the role of your early milk, known as *colostrum*, which is in your breasts during pregnancy and after birth. The World Health Organization calls colostrum "baby's first immunization" because of the many immune factors it contains (WHO 2001). These are especially important to your baby during her first weeks outside the protection of your womb, when she is most vulnerable to infection and illness.

Dairy farmers know that the newborn calf deprived of colostrum is a dead calf, because calves are born with little to no inborn protection from illness. What they need in order to survive comes from their mother's colostrum. To protect their newborn calves, farmers move heaven and earth to make sure the calves get colostrum. We humans receive enough protection from illness and infection before birth to survive without colostrum, as many of us who did not receive colostrum as babies can attest. But although we can live without it, quality of life suffers. A newborn who does not receive her mother's colostrum is a newborn at risk.

Immune factors (macrophages, leukocytes, secretory IgA, and more) in both your colostrum and your mature milk bind microbes and prevent them from entering your baby's delicate tissues. They kill microorganisms and block inflammation. They also promote normal growth of your baby's thymus, an organ devoted solely to developing normal immune function. The thymus in a baby who is fed nonhuman milks is subnormal in size, on average only about half the size of the thymus of an exclusively breastfed baby (Hanson 2004). The immune factors of human milk do not provide breastfed babies with an "extra" boost to their immune system. Human milk is the biological norm—what your baby's body needs and expects at birth. The sad reality is that babies who don't breastfeed suffer from immune-system deficiencies (Labbok, Clark, and Goldman 2004).

Human milk is even more important to at-risk babies. Premature babies who are formula fed take longer to tolerate oral feedings and are six to twenty times more likely to develop necrotizing enterocolitis, a potentially fatal bowel disease (AAP 2005b). Babies born with PKU, a metabolic disorder, lose an average of fourteen IQ points if they are fed formula before their disorder is discovered (Riva et al. 1996). Babies born with cystic fibrosis tend to develop symptoms earlier, grow more slowly, and develop more respiratory infections if they are fed any formula at all (Holliday et al. 1991). Babies with cardiac problems have longer hospital stays and have more problems gaining weight if they miss out on mother's milk (Combs and Marino 1993). Bottom line, for a baby's immune system to function normally, he needs mother's milk.

NORMAL DIGESTIVE HEALTH

Human milk also plays a unique role in digestive health. A newborn's digestive system is sterile and immature at birth and needs help in creating the right environment for digestion and normal development. Right from the start, colostrum creates this normal environment in your baby's digestive system by encouraging the growth of the good bacteria (*bifidus flora*). This good bacteria is responsible for the mild odor of a breastfed baby's stools. A normal gut environment discourages the growth of harmful bacteria and helps a baby's immune system develop properly. If even a small amount of formula or other foods are given, this changes the gut flora so that within twenty-four hours, it resembles that of an adult, which is more vulnerable to harmful bacteria and infection. This is one reason why the Ad Council campaign emphasized exclusive breastfeeding. Once the baby is back to an exclusive human milk diet, it takes two to four weeks for the gut flora to return to normal.

One of the most important functions of colostrum is to seal your newborn's gut to prevent harmful bacteria from sticking to it and penetrating. The junctions between the cells of your baby's intestinal tract are much more open at birth than they will be even several weeks later. While these junctions are open, your baby is vulnerable to allergy triggers (antigens) passing through the gut membranes and causing sensitization. Introducing foreign proteins too early, such as those found in cow's milk and soy-based formulas, can lead to allergy or food intolerance during the first year (Høst 1991).

There are other properties of your milk that are important to your baby's digestive health. For example, growth factors in your milk help your baby's gut to mature more quickly, help the intestinal mucous lining to grow and develop, and strengthen your baby's intestinal barrier. Because a newborn makes few digestive enzymes, human milk provides the bulk of those needed (amylase and bile salts). There are also at least two antioxidants in breast milk that discourage inflammation (Hanson 2004). All of these components help your baby develop a normal digestive system. Anything less can lead to digestive problems.

YOUR BABY'S BRAIN

Breastfeeding is also good for your baby's brain development. One large study of 14,660 babies in the United Kingdom found that babies who were not breastfed were 30 percent more likely to have gross motor delays at nine months than babies who received even some mother's milk and 40 percent more likely to be developmentally delayed than babies exclusively breastfed for at least four months (Sacker, Quigley, and Kelly 2006). A major landmark study in Belarus of 17,046 children found that those children who were breastfed as infants had significantly higher scores on the Wechsler Abbreviated Scales of Intelligence and higher teacher ratings in reading, writing, and math at age six and a half than their counterparts who were not breastfed (Kramer et al. 2008).

Why would this be? One possibility is that your milk has the right mix of fatty acids that are important for your baby's developing brain—especially the omega-3 fatty acid DHA. Yes, this has recently been added to formula. But the problem is that researchers are not entirely sure about the optimal amount, something breastfeeding mothers don't need to worry about. In addition, breastfeeding involves *you*. It's not just a matter of delivering a better product in an attractive package. As you interact with your baby, and respond to her needs, you are giving her just what she needs for her brain to thrive.

Accept No Substitutes

Every few years, the formula companies come up with another "new" ingredient to make formula "more like mother's milk." But what they don't tell you is that vital, living parts of human milk could never survive the canning process, so they will always be missing from formula. And even with the latest new ingredient, there are hundreds of other ingredients in human milk still absent from formula. Some of these ingredients science hasn't even identified yet! Our lack of knowledge is reason enough to avoid man-made substitutes unless absolutely necessary. Even without knowing all the components of human milk, the breastfed baby wins. Breastfeeding is the original no-brainer.

Health Outcomes for You

Our focus up until now has been on your baby. But breastfeeding is also the biological norm for you, and there are negative health outcomes for mothers who don't breastfeed. Moms who don't breastfeed have greater incidence of postpartum hemorrhage, osteoporosis, cardiovascular disease, metabolic syndrome (the precursor to type 2 diabetes), and cancers of the breast, uterus, and ovaries (AAP 2005b; Ram et al. 2008; Schwarz et al. 2009). After birth, mothers who do not breastfeed experience a rapid shift in hormonal levels. Breastfeeding provides a gradual postpartum hormonal shift that can make your transition to motherhood smoother and easier. In chapter 2, we discuss how the hormones of breastfeeding make new motherhood less stressful and bring you and your baby closer. Anything less than exclusive breastfeeding also means a significantly faster return to fertility after birth (AAP 2005b).

Breastfeeding can even impact your financial health. Formula costs a minimum of US$1,200 during your baby's first year. And depending on the type you use and what your baby can tolerate, it could cost you as much as two to three times that amount. This estimate does not include the cost of feeding equipment and extra health care costs, as babies on nonhuman milk tend to be sick more often and more severely (Cunningham, Jelliffe, and Jelliffe 1991). In 1999 dollars, on average, formula-fed babies are estimated to incur US$300–$400 in extra health care costs during their first year of life (Ball and Wright 1999). If you work outside the home, using formula can mean more days off from work to care for a sick child. Any way you look at it, not breastfeeding is expensive.

We're hoping you find this information motivating. Breastfeeding is much more than a lifestyle choice or a nice "touchy-feely" option. It is well worth it for both you and your baby, even if it's tough at first. When we hear the expression "the best things in life are free," one of the first things that comes to mind for us is breastfeeding.

How to Use This Book

This book is organized in two parts. Part 1 explains each of the seven natural laws of breastfeeding and how they work. We will walk with you down the road of normal breastfeeding. Also included in this journey is an explanation of what can happen when the laws are not followed. In chapter 8, we'll also discuss the forces that interfere with the laws and what you can do to counter them.

Part 2 helps you apply the laws to common breastfeeding challenges. It also includes helpful hints on how to fit breastfeeding into your daily life as well as what to do when normal breastfeeding isn't possible. We include specific information on how to find personal help, as a book can never be a substitute for the one-on-one help of a lactation professional. We also have additional information and resources available on our website (www.breastfeedingmadesimple.com). We will refer you to our site throughout the book. This new edition also includes an index to help you locate more easily the information you need about a particular concern.

Regarding our choice of words, we recognize that babies come in two sexes. To acknowledge this while avoiding awkward constructions like "he/she" throughout, we have alternately referred to babies as "he" or "she" in every other chapter.

Finally, our main purpose for writing this book is to help you meet your breastfeeding goals. To do this, we try to strip away the confusion that often accompanies breastfeeding. By focusing on breastfeeding's most basic principles (rather than a complicated list of "rules"), we hope you will find it easier to relax and enjoy your baby. We want your breastfeeding experience to be as simple and joyful as it was meant to be.

PART I

The Laws

CHAPTER 1

Your Baby's Birth

Law 1: *Babies and Mothers Are Hardwired to Breastfeed*

We come into a room where a woman is in the last stages of labor. With a final push, the baby is freed from her mother's body. Immediately after she is born, she is placed on her mother's belly. She lies tummy down and has a chance to get used to the world around her—to breathe on her own, to get used to the louder sounds of the outside world, to adjust to the light. While she is on her mother's belly, she is reassured by her mother's familiar smell and the sound of her voice.

After she has had a while to adjust to the world on the outside, the new baby begins to move purposefully. Pushing with her feet, she slowly moves her way up her mother's body. She travels by her own efforts, slowly but surely, toward her mother's breast. She is encouraged by the sound of Mom's voice and by her smell. When the baby reaches her destination, head bobbing, she opens her mouth, attaches to the breast, and begins to suckle.

Your Baby's Hardwiring

These extraordinary reflex behaviors that allow newborns to move to the breast unaided and to attach are something few of us have seen.

In a more typical scenario, as soon as the baby is born, she is whisked away by an efficient hospital staff. They immediately clean, check, and weigh her, and in some hospitals, put drops in her eyes. It is loud and bright and cold. She begins to cry. Welcome to the world!

While the second scenario is still common, the first is becoming standard practice in more and more places. When mothers and babies are kept skin to skin in the first hour or two after birth, most healthy babies demonstrate the instinctive behaviors that move them to the breast and allow them to attach on their own (Matthieson et al. 2001). And this brings us to Law 1: *Babies and mothers are hardwired to breastfeed.*

"Hardwiring" is a term that neuroscientists use to refer to reflexes and instincts that are built in to your and your baby's bodies and brains. In terms of Law 1, what this means is that babies are born with reflexes and instincts that urge them on to find and suckle at their mothers' breasts. (We'll get to the mother's hardwiring a little later.) Human newborns have this in common with mammals of other species. If you have ever watched a mother cat with a litter of kittens, you have seen the little kittens groping along, trying to get next to their mother. Even though they can't see yet, they use their other senses to gravitate toward their mothers and attach to their nipples, where they find food, comfort, and warmth. This instinctual movement is, in fact, essential for their survival. Doesn't it make sense that human babies would also have that capability? And doesn't it make sense for you to take advantage of it? (If you would like to see this remarkable capability for yourself, we've put a video clip of the "breast crawl" on www. breastfeedingmadesimple.com.)

Newborns' Inborn Feeding Behaviors

We'd like to help you use the inborn breastfeeding reflexes and behaviors that your baby already has. That your baby has these built-in instincts to help her breastfeed is good news. The bad news is that these reflexes and behaviors can be interrupted, short-circuited, or misinterpreted. Not many mothers even know they exist. But even if you've gotten off to a rough start, you can use your baby's built-in responses to get back on track.

The Remarkable Newborn

Newborns can do some pretty amazing things. The ground-breaking work of Dr. Suzanne Colson, a British midwife and researcher, describes in detail the newborn's feeding behaviors and provides tantalizing clues to what appear to be inborn breastfeeding behaviors in mothers, too. As part of her research, Dr. Colson videotaped forty mothers and babies during ninety-three breastfeeding sessions during the first month postpartum and analyzed their movements. She discovered that many of the reflexes triggered during a newborn neurological exam play key roles in breastfeeding. For example, the *stepping reflex* (which makes a newborn held upright appear to walk) occurs when the soles of a baby's feet brush against a firm surface. This reflex was long thought to be unnecessary, but Dr. Colson found that a newborn uses this reflex to push herself to the breast. Dr. Colson identified, in total, twenty *primitive neonatal reflexes,* all of which help a baby breastfeed (Colson, Meek, and Hawdon 2008). Some of these reflexes move baby to the breast, and some help baby attach to and get milk from the breast. And the key to triggering these inborn feeding behaviors is the feel of the mother's body against the front of the baby's chin, torso, hips, and feet.

Dr. Colson also made the remarkable discovery that, like hamsters and puppies, our babies feed best on their tummies and with gravity helping. When mothers in her study leaned back into semi-reclined feeding positions and each newborn was laid tummy down on her mother's body, breastfeeding went much more smoothly. When mothers sat upright or lay on their sides, gravity pulled their babies away and the same inborn feeding behaviors that made breastfeeding work well when babies were tummy down sometimes worked against breastfeeding.

Dr. Colson's work reveals clues to the human version of what is called with other mammals a *feeding sequence.* Pick a mammal—any mammal. Now picture a baby of that species being born. What does it do? Marine mammals make their way to the surface, breathe, then find Mama and nurse. Pouched mammals, born so early that their limbs aren't fully developed, wriggle to the pouch, crawl in, and attach to a teat. Foals, lambs, and baby giraffes struggle to their feet and stagger to Mama's udder. Puppies and kittens and piglets all maneuver themselves to a teat. Whatever mammal you chose, we're sure you can picture its babies making their way to their food source (perhaps with some gentle encouragement from their mothers) in a feeding sequence that is standard for that species. Not surprisingly, human infants, too, have a feeding sequence. But in humans it is often disrupted by clothing, infant seats, cribs, even by the well-meaning parent who thinks the baby's abrupt tumble from shoulder toward chest is accidental and needs to be halted. The first step in working with your baby's feeding sequence is simply recognizing it for what it is.

HOW YOUR BABY FINDS THE BREAST

A baby's senses play a vital role as she makes her journey to the breast after birth.

Your baby knows your voice, scent, and face. Pediatrician Marshall Klaus and clinical social worker Phyllis Klaus documented in their book, *Your Amazing Newborn*, what your baby can do right after birth. From her first moments, a healthy full-term newborn will make eye contact, will turn toward her mother's voice, and can recognize her mother's scent (Klaus and Klaus 2000). Using his Neonatal Behavior Assessment Scale, pediatrician and author T. Berry Brazelton found that newborn babies will turn toward the sound of their mothers' voices and even prefer that voice to others talking at the same time (Brazelton and Nugent 1995). Research indicates that newborns find the breast by using their sense of smell. They recognize their own mother's voice (Bushnell, Sai, and Mullin 1989), respond more distinctly to their own mother's face (Fifer and Moon 1994), and, if separated from their mother, use a very distinct *separation distress call* to locate her (Christensson et al. 1995).

Your unique scent helps your new baby find you. Her sense of touch (on her chest, cheek, chin, and palate) tells her she is close to the breast. Her body position also tells her when her food source is near. Her senses help orient her toward the breast and help her breastfeed.

The role of hunger and thirst. After the first feeding, biochemistry motivates your baby to self-attach. The first and most obvious biochemical reaction is your baby's level of hunger and thirst. When a baby's blood sugar drops, she starts acting hungry. First, she may awaken from sleep. She puts her hands to her mouth, perhaps chewing or sucking on the back of her hand (Klaus and Klaus 2000). Finally, she will start to cry. As a mother, we encourage you to become aware of your baby's feeding cues, especially the early cues, so you can respond to her before she becomes distressed. As we'll discuss in several chapters of this book, it is often difficult to get a screaming baby calmed down enough to breastfeed. And having both of you upset is not ideal when you and your baby are learning to breastfeed in the early days.

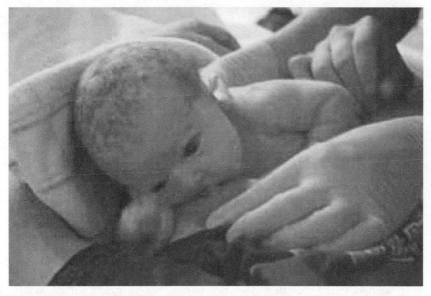

From birth, healthy babies have reflexes that allow them to make their own way to the breast. (© Prue Carr, used with permission)

The role of reflexes. As mentioned earlier, babies have many reflexes that help them breastfeed, including a stepping reflex that they use to push their way up to the breast after birth. They also *root*, meaning that when one cheek is touched, they turn toward whatever is touching them (often, the mother's breast), open their mouths, and drop their tongues in anticipation of breastfeeding.

Your baby's responses to the breast. Suckling at the breast calms your baby and can lead to a feeling of fullness. Often, but not always, once a baby feels full, she pulls off the breast and becomes sleepy. Suckling and skin-to-skin contact also release the hormone oxytocin and other substances that relax her. These hormones turn off hunger's stress responses in your baby and promote emotional attachment with you, as we'll describe in chapter 2. Breastfeeding helps your baby connect being close to you with feeling good. The hormones and physical closeness involved in breastfeeding are part of nature's plan to create a strong mother-baby relationship. Mothers and babies can become close without breastfeeding, but it requires more conscious effort.

Are Mothers Hardwired, Too?

While your baby has lots of hardwiring to help her breastfeed, mothers often wonder about themselves. Many mothers ask, "If breastfeeding is so 'natural,' why am I having problems?" After all, cats do it. Mice do it. Even kangaroos do it. Yet in our complex, high-tech world, many human mothers have a hard time making it work.

Maternal Instincts

It's important to clarify what we mean by instincts. Mothers do indeed come wired with certain *predispositions*, or tendencies, toward specific behaviors. But that does not mean that you will automatically know what to do. When it comes to hardwiring, your baby has an advantage, because her intellect can't get in her way.

YOUR HARDWIRING

Your body is designed to respond to your baby. As you hold your baby, your skin temperature goes up or down, depending on your baby's temperature. In other words, your body helps modulate your baby's body temperature. Your nipples are sensitive and become erect to your baby's touch, making it easier for your baby to locate your breasts.

Breastfeeding releases the hormone oxytocin into your bloodstream, which makes you want to be close to your baby. When your oxytocin levels are elevated, you feel the urge to stroke, touch, and soothe your baby. Oxytocin also causes your breasts to release milk. As you'll see in chapter 2, oxytocin encourages mothers and babies to be more open to one another and to form close relationships (Uvnäs-Moberg 1998, 2003). As Dr. Colson discovered when she analyzed the movements of mothers and babies breastfeeding, when you are relaxed and in sync with your baby, your instincts trigger behaviors that help your baby breastfeed. She called these "sequential patterns of instinctual maternal behaviors" and wrote that mothers with at least one hand free in semireclining breastfeeding positions spontaneously stroked their babies feet, which released reflexes in the baby that triggered lip and tongue movements. As she writes, "mothers appeared to trigger instinctively the right reflex at the right time" (Colson, Meek, and Hawdon 2008, 446).

YOUR BRAIN CAN OVERRIDE YOUR HARDWIRING

Because human mothers have large brains, their natural responses can be easily overridden, despite biological triggers. Along with biological responses that encourage breastfeeding, mothers also have free will. Human mothers' instincts are not like those of, say, bees. When bees respond to an instinct, they have no choice but to follow predetermined behaviors. In contrast, humans and some other primates do have a choice. Our bodies may encourage us to behave in a certain way, but we decide whether or not to follow the urge. Our urges can also be overridden by our beliefs or our cultural norms. We'll discuss this effect in more detail in chapter 8.

WHAT YOU LEARN AFFECTS BREASTFEEDING

The bottom line for you is that while breastfeeding is natural (it's one of the things that makes us mammals), breastfeeding instruction affects your behavior. Your body may provide you with cues about what to do. For instance, when you hear your baby cry, your milk may let down. When your baby begins to root or fuss, you may feel a strong urge to pick your baby up and even put her in a position that will allow her to breastfeed, noting that this position seems soothing. But if you use your intellect to breastfeed and follow instructions from others, this sometimes makes breastfeeding more difficult, leaving you with no idea what to do next. If this is you, be kind to yourself. Take a deep breath and give yourself permission to try some different approaches.

How Mothers Learn to Breastfeed

When mothers have breastfeeding problems, many admit to either feeling "stupid" or concerned that their maternal instincts are faulty. But learning to breastfeed need not be difficult or require lots of instruction. Friends, family, and even health professionals can make breastfeeding sound so complicated that many women worry that they won't be able to do it. This is often a case of too much information given with the wrong emphasis.

Our perspective might strike you as odd, since this is an instructional book about breastfeeding. But stick with us here. Mothers in developed countries have huge amounts of information available on breastfeeding. There are classes, videos, and tons of books. Websites offer a full range of information on everything from common problems to the more obscure. Mothers now have more "expert" information on breastfeeding than ever before.

We are not trying to malign that information in any way. In fact, we've written our share of words about breastfeeding ourselves. But if reading breastfeeding articles or books were enough, the United States should have one of the highest breastfeeding rates in the world, which is far from the reality. Instead, this glut of well-meaning information has managed to make quite a few mothers anxious and confused about breastfeeding.

A different way to think about this is to consider how mothers throughout human history managed to breastfeed without all of the information that we have now. When breastfeeding was the norm, girls learned about breastfeeding as they were growing up by seeing women actually doing it. Dr. Peter Hartmann, a well-known breastfeeding researcher, makes this point well with this anecdote that he shared at a breastfeeding conference some years ago. He asked a young Australian Aboriginal mother, "When did you learn about breastfeeding?" She answered, "I have always known how to breastfeed."

"Head" Knowledge vs. "Body" Knowledge

In Western cultures, we have replaced that kind of "doing" knowledge with book knowledge. And therein lies the challenge. In order to simplify breastfeeding, we want you to understand the built-in mechanisms, or "natural laws," that make breastfeeding easier for you and your baby. In the process, we also want to avoid giving you lots of "head" knowledge about breastfeeding.

The work of Dr. Christina Smillie, a pediatrician and board-certified lactation consultant, provides helpful insights into a different approach to breastfeeding. Using Dr. Smillie's term, we prefer to think of breastfeeding as a *right-brained* activity (Smillie 2008). What do we mean by that? Think of *left-brained* instructions as head knowledge. Right-brained learning yields heart or body knowledge. To illustrate this difference, think about riding a bike. Did you learn by reading about it, taking a class, or talking to other people about it? Or did you learn by just getting on a bike and doing it?

Mothers, Brains, and Breastfeeding

Mothers are influenced in many ways. Mothers and babies have physiological responses that draw them to each other, that encourage them to look at each other, touch each other, and interact. Much of this behavior is guided by the right side of the brain. This is the side that has to do with affect or emotion. In fact, some characterize mothers' and babies' interactions as being like a dance. But rather than being choreographed by others, the movements of this dance come from within, with the actions of one influencing the actions of the other.

How Overthinking Breastfeeding Can Hinder You

A problem with the heavily left-brained, instructionally oriented way that many mothers learn to breastfeed is that it doesn't allow mother and baby to take advantage of their natural responses (Smillie 2008). So much breastfeeding education focuses on all the things the mother must do to get the baby to breastfeed, which ignores the baby's responses. Many of the breastfeeding books and classes also emphasize using specific upright or side-lying feeding positions, which can make breastfeeding more difficult during the early weeks. That type of instruction can be helpful to solve a particular problem, but it can be a definite drawback when one technique or strategy is applied to all mothers—a one-size-fits-all approach to breastfeeding. It also discourages mothers and babies from using their hardwiring. Worse still, this kind of education can encourage mothers to tune out their natural responses or to violate their instincts. It can be upsetting for all who are involved, sometimes creating a crisis where none existed before.

Another problem with highly instructional, left-brained approaches is that they can leave some mothers feeling incompetent, because it feels as if there is a list of ten thousand things they need to remember. British researcher Suzanne Colson notes that when a mother relies too much on her left brain during breastfeeding, it can actually inhibit the release of those hormones, such as oxytocin, that can relax her and help her fall in love with her baby (Colson, Meek, and Hawdon 2008).

Breastfeeding the Right-Brained Way

Now let's get more specific. How exactly do you use a right-brained approach to breastfeed your baby?

BREASTFEEDING AS A RELATIONSHIP

First, take some deep breaths and let go of those worries about doing things "wrong." Instead of thinking of breastfeeding as a skill you need to master, or a measure of your worth as a mother, think about breastfeeding as primarily a relationship. As you spend time with your baby, you'll be more adept at reading her cues. As you hold her (and we encourage you to hold your baby a lot), your baby will be more comfortable in seeking your breast. Breastfeeding will flow naturally out of your affectionate relationship.

When Dr. Colson analyzed mothers' and babies' movements during breastfeeding, she discovered that some simple body dynamics made a huge difference in how smoothly early breastfeeding went. Here are some specific things you can do.

Start with a calm baby. One mistake that many women make is to wait to try breastfeeding until their babies are crying. Think about yourself. Do you learn best when you are upset? Probably not.

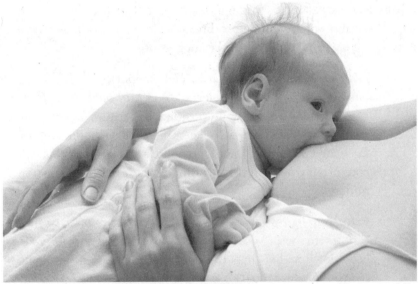

In a laid-back breastfeeding position like this, your arms are free to cuddle your baby, making it easy to relax and enjoy your time together.

There's another reason to start with a calm baby. This one is based on pure physics. When your baby is crying, note where her tongue is. In most cases, it is on the roof of her mouth—unless she is lowering it to take a deep breath before screaming again. If her tongue is raised, how is she going to get your breast in her mouth? When your baby is calmer, she is in the best frame of mind to both learn and feed.

Watch for early feeding cues. These cues include rooting (turning her head when something touches her cheek) or hand-to-mouth (see chapter 4 for more on this). It's obviously better if you can catch your calm baby at the first sign of hunger, so take note of when she starts smacking her lips or putting her hands to her mouth, even if she's in a light sleep. This is an ideal time to try breastfeeding.

Sometimes you don't catch your baby in the early hunger stages (such as when you're sound asleep!) and have to deal with a baby who is upset. And some babies go from a little hungry to very hungry in a really short time. To calm your baby, offer the breast. If this doesn't work, don't force the issue or you'll end up with a real problem, like a baby who associates her time at the breast with frustration. If this happens, calm your baby before breastfeeding by holding, swaying, rocking, or walking. Then try these suggestions:

- *Lean back and get comfortable.* Well-supported semireclined positions are sometimes referred to as *laid-back breastfeeding*. This may be the same position you use to watch your favorite television show. Make sure you have good support for your back, neck, shoulders, and arms so that you can comfortably relax in this position for at least thirty to sixty minutes.

- *Place your baby, tummy down, between your breasts.* You can do this with your baby dressed or you can strip your baby down to her diaper. Then make your breast available to her. You can do this by unbuttoning your shirt from the bottom or top, pulling your shirt up past your breasts, wearing a roomy shirt that can cover you both or, in the privacy of your own home, simply not wearing anything on top. Your chest is a very calming place for your baby. She can hear your voice and your heartbeat. She can smell you and get the feeling of your skin. Talk with her and make eye contact to establish a right-brained connection that will bring you closer to your baby.

- *Follow your baby's lead.* When a calm baby lies tummy down on her mother's semireclined body, this triggers instinctive breast-seeking behaviors such as head-bobbing and movements toward the breast. If she is lying between your breasts, she probably won't need much help. Encourage her explorations with your voice. Babies can't understand your words at this age, but they can understand your tone of voice. When a baby hears a calm, encouraging voice, she feels emboldened to try new things. Use the other tips listed below and in chapter 3 to help use her hardwiring to latch on to the breast with a minimum of frustration.

Play while you learn to breastfeed. Play is something that is largely absent in the mothers that we see. Often, especially if they are having problems, these mothers are distraught, worried about doing things wrong, and feeling like they are failing this first "crucial test" of motherhood. If you're feeling frustrated, we'd like to encourage you to look at this another way. Focus on your relationship with your baby and consider breastfeeding as a part of this larger whole. As we described earlier, breastfeeding will flow naturally out of your affectionate relationship. For instance, your baby may try to latch on when not particularly hungry but when she is trying out her new skill. These practice times are good for your relationship and will serve you well when she is hungry.

Can you see how this approach differs from one that emphasizes picking up your baby only when she is screaming or seeing your baby as a blank slate who relies on you to do everything right? Having worked with lots of mothers and babies over the years, we've always been amazed at how well breastfeeding can work when mothers and babies are ready and responsive to each other.

USING OTHER ASPECTS OF YOUR BABY'S HARDWIRING

When we say that babies are hardwired to breastfeed (Law 1), we mean that they are born with natural reflexes that help them find and suckle at their mothers' breasts. This includes the instinctive drive to find your breasts, as we discussed earlier. Here are some other ways you can take advantage of your baby's hardwiring.

Make sure baby's body is not twisted and there are no gaps between you. This is easy when you are leaning back, as gravity does most of the work of keeping your baby's body pressed against yours.

This also means you don't have to support your baby's weight with your arms, which makes feedings much more relaxing and restful.

If baby seems uncomfortable, adjust her body position or your angle of recline. When your baby is lying tummy down on your body, she can approach the breast in many different ways. She can lie on your body lengthwise or diagonally, or she can lie across your breasts, which may be most comfortable for you after a cesarean birth. And there are lots of variations of these positions. Suzanne Colson has noticed that before taking the breast, some babies like to assume positions similar to those they used in the womb (Colson 2005). She says the best position is that in which mother and baby fit together like two pieces of a puzzle. No matter what position you and your baby use during feedings, she will feel more secure and relaxed if she feels your steadying warmth against her whole body.

The touch of the baby's chin against your body triggers a wide-open mouth. For a good, deep latch, babies need to open wide while attaching to the breast, and your baby's hardwiring can help with this. (We'll describe this in more detail in chapter 3.) When a baby feels this touch against her chin, it's as though you are speaking her language. When your baby lies tummy down, as she opens her mouth wide over your breast, gravity helps to pull her on farther, for a deep, comfortable latch. Some babies get on the breast more comfortably if their mothers help to shape the breast for them, which is fine. When breastfeeding is a relationship, both people play an important role. There's no reason your baby has to go to the breast all by herself. And remember, it's fine to experiment as there is more than one right way to breastfeed. The more you do what works for both you and your baby, the easier and more automatic breastfeeding will become.

The drinking position: Head back, chin forward. Rebecca Glover, RM, IBCLC, a midwife and lactation consultant from Australia, notes another aspect to babies' hardwiring. When a baby gets ready to feed, she instinctively throws her head back and thrusts her chin forward. Glover points out that we adults also do this when we're thirsty and drink fast (think about how you chug a tall, cool glass of water on a hot day) (Glover and Wiessinger 2008).

To understand why babies do this, put your chin to your chest and try to swallow. See how difficult that is? To keep your throat open for drinking, it works best to have your head slightly tilted back. It's the same for babies. However your baby is positioned at the breast, avoid pushing on her head and be sure she can tilt her head slightly back into this instinctive feeding position. This will make drinking much easier for her.

Feeling the breast in the comfort zone. This point is covered in detail in chapter 3 but deserves a mention here. There is a special place deep in your baby's mouth that triggers active suckling. When you achieve a deep latch and your nipple reaches this "comfort zone," not only is breastfeeding comfortable for you, but your baby's hardwiring is triggered to help her feed well and actively. When she feels your breast there, she gets a better milk flow and breastfeeding is easier. A shallower latch results in a slower milk flow, which can cause many babies to fall asleep quickly or "tune out" at the breast.

After birth, keep mother and baby skin to skin. If you are reading this during your pregnancy, make arrangements to stay skin to skin with your baby for that first hour or two after birth if at all possible. This is one of the easiest ways to trigger your baby's hardwiring. Because you will probably not be in a state of mind to take charge right after giving birth, it is best to arrange for your partner or labor support person to be responsible for talking to the staff about your wishes. If you and your baby are healthy, the birth staff should be expected to honor this request, even if they are unfamiliar with babies' instinctive behaviors. This is one easy and effective way to help get breastfeeding off to a good start.

Using your baby's hardwiring, especially when you're skin to skin (see chapter 2), will help you tune in to your baby's cues more easily. You will spend more time touching, stroking, and talking to your baby, which helps her neurological development and increases your milk production. With practice, you will begin to feel like the real expert on your baby. And it will help you see your baby as competent, too. You won't need outside experts to tell you that you're doing a good job, because you'll be able to see it with your own eyes. And watching your baby thrive is the best part of all.

When the System Breaks Down

Babies are born knowing how to make their way to the breast, but there are factors that can interfere with this natural process. Knowing this can help you get a good start.

Birth Interventions and Separation

Research has found that some of the choices made during and after birth can temporarily affect your baby's inborn feeding behaviors. In one study of eighty mothers and babies, two factors were found to short-circuit, in the short term, a baby's breast-seeking reflexes:

- the use during labor of Demerol (meperidine), a narcotic pain reliever

- a short separation of mother and baby for cleaning and weighing before the first breastfeeding

Not one of the babies who experienced both of these factors attached to the breast and breastfed well during the first two hours after birth. Of the babies who experienced only one of these factors, about half breastfed well in their first two hours. Of the babies who experienced neither—no separation after birth and no Demerol during labor—all but one breastfed well during this time (Righard and Alade 1990).

Because birth is tiring for both you and your baby, after this first two hours, most babies go into a long stretch of sleep. Missing this first feeding decreases the number of total breastfeedings you can fit in during the first twenty-four hours. The overall number of breastfeedings this first day can affect how long it takes for your milk to increase and whether or not your baby develops exaggerated newborn jaundice (see chapter 4). Missing this first feeding is definitely not enough to compromise breastfeeding (legions of mothers and babies whose first breastfeeding was delayed can attest to this), but it puts you and your baby at higher risk for problems and complications. By setting up the right conditions during these first two hours and encouraging baby's feeding behaviors after birth, using this first law can help you avoid potential problems down the line.

Also, it's important to know that this is not the only study that has found that labor medications and birth interventions can affect breast-feeding. One study found an association between the use of several pain medications given to mothers in labor with more crying, a decrease in breast-seeking behaviors, and less suckling in their newborns (Ransjö-Arvidson et al. 2001). Another study found that the babies of mothers who received an epidural during labor were less alert, less able to orient themselves, and had less organized movements as compared with babies whose mothers received no pain medication during labor (Sepkoski et al. 1992). Surprisingly, researchers found that these differences continued throughout the babies' first month of life.

Birth interventions, such as roughly sucking the mucus from the nose and mouth and the use of forceps or vacuum extraction, can also affect a baby's willingness to breastfeed after birth. And although it is beyond the scope of this book to comprehensively cover the effects of birth interventions on breastfeeding, we encourage you to learn more. To this end, we recommend the book *Impact of Birthing Practices on Breastfeeding* by Linda J. Smith (2010), which is listed in our Resources section at the end of this book.

Hospital Routines

Many of the routines followed in hospitals today were created during a time when formula feeding was the norm. From the hospital's standpoint, it made no sense to keep mothers and babies together when most babies were fed nonhuman milks. On the contrary, the focus was on helping the mother to "get her rest," and limiting her contact with her baby was central to that.

GETTING YOUR REST

The issue of getting your rest is obviously legitimate, especially after a long or difficult labor. But no one should ever have to choose between getting her rest and feeding her baby! In breastfeeding-friendly hospitals, mothers are helped to get their rest while they breastfeed. In one hospital in central Illinois, the lactation consultant trains the staff nurses to help mothers feed their babies while lying down. This allows mothers to nap and feed at the same time. One study, not surprisingly, found that women who breastfeed lying down report less fatigue than women who breastfeed sitting up (Milligan, Flenniken, and Pugh 1996). Also, adjustable hospital beds make it easy to use semireclined, laid-back feeding positions, which eliminate the need for you to support your baby's weight during feedings, making feeding more relaxing and restful.

TASK FOCUS VS. HUMAN NEEDS

In some institutions, mother-baby separation and "sanitary procedures" are still considered more important than a mother and her baby getting to know each other. Sometimes this process is interrupted for no other reason than that the mother and baby are not conforming to the hospital's sense of time. Perhaps the hospital staff needs the room for another mother. Or maybe allowing the mother and baby to just "be" doesn't appeal to the hospital staff's sense of aesthetics or efficiency. In these cases, the justification doesn't really hold up. As we mentioned earlier, when the baby is immediately whisked away to be cleaned, measured, and so on, that quiet receptive period after birth is lost. When mother and baby are separated after birth and before the first feeding, babies' inborn feeding behaviors can be sabotaged or suppressed, making breastfeeding more difficult.

Medical Condition of the Mother or Baby

Sometimes mothers or babies are not able to start breastfeeding right away because one or both of them have a medical condition that needs to be attended to immediately. The mother's and baby's health take precedence over getting to know each other. For example, if a mother is hemorrhaging, she needs immediate attention. If a baby isn't breathing or has some other emergency medical issue, that needs to be dealt with at once.

Some mothers who have had surgical births may also be separated from their babies immediately after birth. However, in many hospitals, mothers are helped to breastfeed right after a cesarean birth, while they are still comfortable and before their pain medication wears off.

If You Get Off to a Difficult Start

If you have somehow gotten off to a bad start, for whatever reason, do not fear. Baby's instinctive breast-seeking behaviors don't disappear immediately after birth, and you can continue using them to make breastfeeding work. Through her practice, Dr. Christina Smillie has found that several months after birth, even if a baby hasn't been breast-feeding or feeding well, these instinctive behaviors remain intact for healthy babies (Smillie 2008). This is great news for mothers and babies who've gotten a rocky start.

IS IT TOO LATE?

We are grateful for the pioneering work of Marshall Klaus and John Kennell in their studies of mother/infant bonding and the impor-tance of that time immediately after birth (Klaus, Kennell, and Klaus 1996). Unfortunately, in actual practice, we've seen this research badly applied. Some mothers truly believe that if they miss that initial time (as many do), then all is lost. This was never supposed to be the message of the bonding research! It's true that the contact immedi-ately after birth can make things easier. However, breastfeeding and bonding with your baby are too critical to your baby's survival and well-being to be given only one chance to work. The good news is that even if you missed that early time together, it is definitely not too late. Babies still know how to attach to the breast. This ability is not limited to the first twenty-four hours after birth. You can help your baby use this amazing ability through your physical closeness with each other and your playful interactions. These will help your baby learn to breastfeed.

Summary

We hope that knowing something about your own and your baby's feeding reflexes and behaviors will help increase your self-confidence as you prepare for breastfeeding. We also hope that if you find early breastfeeding challenging, something as simple as leaning back to breastfeed can help make your early weeks of breastfeeding easier and more relaxing.

CHAPTER 2

The Power of Touch: Why Holding Your Baby Matters

Law 2: *Mother's Body Is the Baby's Natural Habitat*

There's nothing that feels quite so right as a mother holding her baby skin to skin. A baby's smell and the feel of a baby's skin are intoxicating. For a baby, too, there is nothing as comforting as his mother's touch. Yet, as universal and as human as these feelings are, there is more to it than that—much more.

That mothers love to touch their babies is nothing new. What is new is our increasing understanding of the power of touch. In fact, in some parts of the world and in some situations, the simple act of a mother holding her baby close has made the difference between life and death.

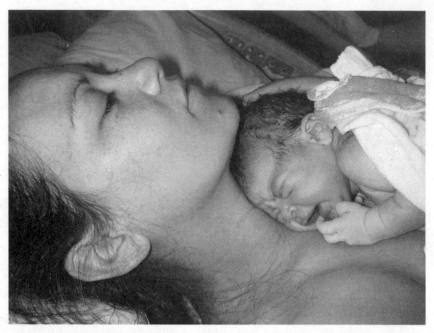

Skin-to-skin contact calms you and your baby. Your touch is vital to his growth and good health. (©2005 Marilyn Nolt, used with permission)

Lactation consultants and other skilled breastfeeding counselors have long known that putting mothers and babies skin to skin can help solve many breastfeeding problems. But now we are beginning to learn why. And the story is a fascinating one.

The Habitat of the Human Newborn

To begin to understand the power of skin-to-skin contact, we must take you on an excursion through mammalian biology. To do this, we draw upon the work of Dr. Nils Bergman, a South African physician who has had remarkable success in decreasing infant mortality in rural Zimbabwe. In the part of the world where Dr. Bergman lived, there was one doctor for every 100,000 people, and those doctors did not have incubators and other technology found in most hospital special-care nurseries (Bergman 2001b). Prior to Dr. Bergman's work, the infant mortality rate for premature babies was a staggering 70 percent. Dr. Bergman discovered that, by wrapping tiny premature babies skin to skin with their mothers twenty-three hours a day (which he calls *Kangaroo Mother Care*), he could use the power of skin-to-skin contact to improve infant survival of the smallest preemies in Zimbabwe from 10 percent to 50 percent (Bergman and Jurisoo 1994). Drs. Rey and Hernandez, both neonatologists in Bogotá, Colombia, developed a similar program with preterm babies in their hospital and had similarly remarkable results (Ludington-Hoe with Golant 1993).

More recently, researchers in India compared Kangaroo Care to standard care in 135 low–birth weight, preterm babies. Their findings are similar to those observed in Africa and Colombia. Babies in Kangaroo Care had more stable oxygen levels and heart rates, cried less and slept more, and were more likely to breastfeed. The mothers indicated that Kangaroo Care made them feel more competent in handling their babies. It also improved their mood and helped them feel closer to their babies. This happened even when the mothers were initially nervous about trying Kangaroo Care (Parmar et al. 2009).

By studying Kangaroo Care (any amount of skin-to-skin contact) and Kangaroo Mother Care (extended skin-to-skin contact), we have learned much about the power of skin-to-skin contact, not just as it benefits preemies, but also as a way to promote normal health and breastfeeding for full-term, healthy newborns. In a study from Iran, researchers found that infants held skin to skin with their mothers for just ten minutes showed significantly fewer signs of pain when they received an injection compared with infants who were not held in Kangaroo Care (Kashaninia et al. 2008).

A Newborn Mammal's Natural Programming

Dr. Bergman is not only a medical doctor; he has also studied animal biology and behavior, and his studies of other species were instrumental in the development of his Kangaroo Mother Care approach. In fact, he uses the biologist's term "habitat" to explain why Kangaroo Mother Care has saved so many babies' lives. *Habitat* is the place where behavior occurs. And a mother's body is a baby's natural habitat, the place where babies breastfeed.

All mammals have behaviors that are programmed into their hard-wiring and vary depending on their habitat or location. Dr. Bergman points out: "Mothers don't breastfeed: babies breastfeed. The mother's body is simply the habitat where the baby feeds" (2001b). It is best to keep mother and baby together right from birth. As we discussed in chapter 1, if a baby is left on his mother's abdomen after a medication-free birth, the newborn makes his way to the breast, finds the nipple, and starts breastfeeding. (If you want to see a video clip of a baby doing this, we have one on www.breastfeedingmadesimple.com.) The baby responds to his mother's scent, her voice, and the feel of her skin. For human infants, breastfeeding and being held close to mother are critical to survival. The behavior, in this case, breastfeeding, is determined by the habitat—baby's closeness to his mother's body.

WHAT HAPPENS WHEN BABIES ARE NOT IN THEIR HABITAT

If a newborn is removed from his habitat (his mother's body), it triggers instincts that can be counterproductive to breastfeeding—and indeed, to life itself. Dr. Bergman explains that in all mammal babies, there are two basic "programs" governed by the part of the brain called the *hindbrain* (2001b). These two programs, defense and nutrition, are keys to our survival. They regulate hormones, nerves, and muscles, affecting the whole body. The problem is that at any given time, only one program can run. If the defense program is running, the body shuts off the nutrition program, and with it, growth. If the nutrition program is running, a baby's defenses are shut down.

Separation, the defense program, and the protest-despair response. For a newborn, separation from his mother throws his body into defense mode. If you separate a human baby (or any other mammal) from his mother, a physical reaction occurs and the baby responds by loudly protesting with a distinctive cry known as the *separation distress call* (Christensson et al. 1995). Biologists call the set of behaviors that occur when babies are removed from their mothers the *protest-despair response.*

When a baby's protest is prolonged and unanswered, the next emotion he experiences is despair. Once this programming has been triggered, a baby is in defense mode, and, to increase the odds of survival, his body begins to shut down, using less energy by decreasing his heart rate, breathing rate, and body temperature. In this mode, every other function is shut down so that little growth is taking place.

When a baby is in this protest phase, his tiny body produces huge amounts of stress hormones, and the baby physically prepares to fight for survival (Michelsson et al. 1996). The stress response is meant to be a short-term response. But when it is "on" all the time, it causes a number of health problems. And that is true for both infants and adults. The stress hormones shut down gut function, digestion, and growth. In fact, Dr. Bergman points out that what are now considered by many medical experts to be the normal ranges of heart rate, body temperature, and stress hormones of preemies separated from their mothers in high-tech nurseries are not normal at all but reflect this protest-despair response (2001b). Interestingly, this same reaction occurs in every mammal that's ever been studied.

If you've ever wondered why some babies have such a hard time being set down and left alone, now you know: a newborn's whole body is set to react intensely to separation from his mother.

When together, the nutrition program promotes growth. In contrast, when a newborn is held skin to skin with his mother, the opposite reaction occurs. Being in his natural habitat (touching his mother's body) stimulates the nutrition program. As Dr. Bergman describes (and as his amazing results with premature babies have demonstrated), when a newborn is in the right habitat (touching his mother), his brain responds by triggering the program for growth. His level of stress hormones decreases by 74 percent (Mooncey 1997). His gut begins to process food (Uvnäs-Moberg et al. 1987; Uvnäs-Moberg 2003). His heart rate and breathing return to normal. If the baby is touching his mother, his physiology is no longer sounding the alarm.

The life-and-death consequences of mother-infant separation were carefully documented by the researchers who eventually developed what is known as *attachment theory*. Psychiatrists Rene Spitz and, later, John Bowlby observed orphans in Europe at the end of World War II who actually died from lack of emotional attachment to a caregiver, even though their physical needs were met. (For more detail on the history of attachment theory, we'd recommend *Our Babies, Ourselves* by Meredith Small [1998] and *A General Theory of Love* by Thomas Lewis, Fari Amini, and Richard Lannon [2000].) That a lack of emotional attachment could lead to death was a radical idea in the 1940s and 1950s. American social sciences were still dominated by behaviorism—an ideology that still, unfortunately, permeates much of today's childrearing advice. Behaviorists maintained that meeting children's physical needs was enough. They considered the idea that children needed affectionate relationships to be absurd. To his credit, Bowlby persisted in his work and gradually changed people's minds.

Not surprisingly, other primates also have a strong drive to be in snuggle contact with their mothers. More than fifty years ago, Harry Harlow conducted a series of experiments in which newborn monkeys had access to both a wire mesh "mother" and a soft, terry-cloth "mother" (Harlow 1959). In some cages one mother had an attached bottle, in other cages, not. No matter which mother provided food, babies spent far more time cuddling on the cloth mother than on the wire mesh mother. Harlow noted that when baby monkeys had no access to a cloth mother, they developed strong attachments to the cloths that lined their cage in ways that reminded him strongly of human childhood attachments to blankets and teddies. Without anything soft to cling to at all, baby monkeys became emotionally disturbed and had difficulty surviving. He noted, "We were impressed by the possibility that, above and beyond the bubbling fountain of breast or bottle, contact comfort might be a very important variable in the development of the infant's affection for the mother" (Harlow 1959, 577).

We're finding that those early experiences have longer-term implications than we ever believed, affecting health throughout the lifespan. For example, an article in a recent edition of the *Journal of the American Medical Association* made a rather remarkable statement: "Adult disease prevention begins with reducing early toxic stress" (Shonkoff, Boyce, and McEwen 2009, 2256). They go on to develop their premise that the quality of early relationships has a profound impact on people's health throughout their lives and reduces the risk of such life-threatening illnesses as cardiovascular disease, metabolic syndrome, and diabetes.

What do these findings mean for you? Quite simply, they mean that what you do now has a long-lasting effect on your baby's future health. As a new mother, you will probably be told that it's important to "train" your baby to be independent. But if you look at this research from the broader perspective of adult health, you will see that the "independence" advice is really quite wrong. When looking at the whole of life, people who are isolated from each other have higher rates of disease and even premature death. From a health standpoint, the goal is not independence, but *interdependence* and having social connections with other people. And if that is true for adults, how much more would it be true for a defenseless newborn?

THE EFFECTS OF SKIN-TO-SKIN CONTACT AND KEEPING MOTHERS AND BABIES TOGETHER AFTER BIRTH

In light of these remarkable differences, is it any wonder that keeping mothers and babies together helps to promote breastfeeding? All of these findings explain why putting a baby back into his natural habitat calms and normalizes his nervous system, making him more receptive to growth-promoting behaviors such as feeding and digestion. Mothers are also less stressed when they are not separated from their babies. In fact, mothers and babies regulate each others physiologic states. Early skin-to-skin contact between mother and baby has also been found to affect how long mothers continue to breastfeed babies, with more skin-to-skin contact after birth linked to more exclusive breastfeeding at hospital discharge (Bramson et al. 2010) and an increased number of months of breastfeeding (Mikiel-Kostyra, Mazur, and Boltruszko 2002). And it can also help solve breastfeeding problems when they occur.

How Skin-to-Skin Contact Works

Scientists have proven that skin-to-skin contact between mother and baby has profound effects on them both. Now let's take a closer look at the reasons.

IF IT FEELS GOOD, OXYTOCIN MUST BE INVOLVED

There is far more to our mental and emotional states than just our hormones. But we also know that our hormones can affect us, sometimes in subtle ways. *Oxytocin*, which comes from the Latin word meaning "swift birth," is both a hormone and a central nervous system neurotransmitter that is released during skin-to-skin contact.

THE ROLES OF OXYTOCIN

Oxytocin has a role in many aspects of human physiology, many of which affect relationships (Uvnäs-Moberg 2003). If you are unfamiliar with oxytocin, here are some examples of when it is released and what it does:

- It is released during orgasm in both men and women.

- It causes the contractions of the uterus during labor (its synthetic form, pitocin, is sometimes given to induce or speed labor).

- It is released when a person experiences warm temperatures, touch, stroking, acupuncture, and massage.

- It is released after a good meal and probably helps explain why so many of our celebrations and rituals that bring people together involve sharing a meal.

- It is directly responsible for the contraction of muscles in the breast, which causes milk release (sometimes called the *let-down* or *milk-ejection reflex*) during breastfeeding (Newton 1978).

Swedish researcher Kerstin Uvnäs-Moberg and her colleagues have been studying oxytocin for many decades, and some of their findings explain why skin-to-skin contact has such far-reaching implications for biology and behavior (Uvnäs-Moberg 2003). For example, here are some of the physical effects of oxytocin and related peptides:

- greater blood flow to the breasts in mothers and to the skin of infants

- increased appetite and greater digestive efficiency

- decreased blood pressure and production of stress hormones, such as cortisol

+ increased ability to learn (i.e., you learn better when you are calm)

+ increased blood sugar and insulin levels

+ increased pain threshold and enhanced wound healing

One interesting property of oxytocin is that, although its direct effect on the body is only minutes long, its long-term effects can last for weeks (Uvnäs-Moberg 1998; 2003). Oxytocin produces physical changes that have also been found to affect mood and behavior. It has a sedating effect, calms mood, decreases anxiety, and increases stable personality traits. It decreases the desire to move around and increases the tolerance of monotony. It increases openness to social direction and bonding with peers. It increases "nesting" behaviors. And it enhances acceptance of offspring and bonding between mother and baby. From what we know of it, oxytocin appears to play a key role in bringing people together and cementing relationships (Uvnäs-Moberg 1998; 2003).

Oxytocin and milk release. During breastfeeding, oxytocin is responsible for the release of milk from the breast, a vital aspect of successful breastfeeding and milk expression. Many women think that milk flow from the breast (either to the baby or to a pump) occurs as a result of suction. Actually, that is not the case. Getting milk from the breast is not like sucking liquid through a straw. With a straw, the stronger you suck, the more liquid you get. With the breast, however, the key to milk flow is triggering a milk release.

When a baby latches on to the breast and begins to suckle, the nerve impulses sent to the mother's brain cause the release of oxytocin in her bloodstream. As in labor, oxytocin causes muscles to contract. But the muscles responsible for milk release are in the breasts. These muscles squeeze the milk-producing glands and actively push the milk toward the nipple while the milk ducts widen. Some mothers feel this as a tingling sensation in their breasts; others feel nothing. Some women leak milk from the other breast when the milk releases; others don't. When you hear your baby swallowing, you know you've had a milk release. A milk release can be triggered by many things: a certain touch at the breast, hearing a baby cry, or even by thinking about your baby. Feelings of tension, anger, or frustration can block it.

During breastfeeding, most mothers have several milk releases without even knowing it (Ramsay et al. 2004). The physical cues from your baby make milk release happen automatically. Your baby is soft; your baby is warm; you love your baby. All of these cues cause your milk to flow. When a mother pumps, these physical cues are missing, so getting a milk release can sometimes be trickier, but there are ways to make this happen. (For more on this, see chapter 9.)

Breastfeeding lowers your stress levels. Some mothers are told by the uninformed that breastfeeding is stressful. Of course, breastfeeding problems can be stressful. But if breastfeeding is going smoothly, the opposite is actually true. While caring for a newborn can most definitely be intense and sometimes stressful (no matter how he is fed), this is unrelated to breastfeeding.

Considering what we know about oxytocin, it's not surprising that research indicates that it is more stressful not to breastfeed than to breastfeed (Uvnäs-Moberg 2003). The extra time spent skin to skin and the subsequent oxytocin release that is a normal part of breastfeeding no doubt play a part in this. Two recent studies of the stress-reducing effects of breastfeeding have found that it lowers the stress response:

- In one study, researchers compared the experiences of women who both breastfed and bottlefed to demonstrate the calming effect of breastfeeding. Researchers assessed each mother's mood before and after breastfeeding and before and after bottlefeeding. Their findings indicated that the mothers in the study were calmer after breastfeeding than after bottlefeeding. This study was significant because it eliminated one of the major problems in comparing breastfeeding and nonbreastfeeding women: the often substantial differences between women who choose one feeding method over the other. Since the same mothers were studied after both breast and bottle, this potentially confounding factor was eliminated (Mezzacappa and Katkin 2002).

- In another study, researchers compared the stress levels of women when they held their babies skin to skin and when they were actually breastfeeding. Skin to skin was good, but breastfeeding was even better. In addition, for about half an hour after breastfeeding, the women were more resistant to stress when the experimenters tried to stress them (Heinrichs et al. 2001).

In summarizing findings from these previous studies, researcher Maureen Groer and her colleagues note that the stress-lowering effects of breastfeeding on mothers are important for infant survival because they incline mothers toward nurturing behaviors and conservation of energy (Groer, Davis, and Hemphill 2002; Groer and Davis 2006).

Other health effects for you. The oxytocin response triggered by both skin-to-skin contact and breastfeeding may have many far-reaching effects on you. It causes a decrease in aggressive and defensive feelings, making you feel more open to the new little "stranger" to whom you have given birth. Oxytocin influences your mood, makes you calmer, and promotes a closer relationship with your baby and your partner (Uvnäs-Moberg 2003). The effects of oxytocin may also help with relationships outside your family. This may be one reason why many breastfeeding mothers love the atmosphere of mothers' groups, where those with high levels of oxytocin gather and befriend one another.

What's even more amazing are the results of two recent studies of older women; these studies found that the stress-reducing aspects of breastfeeding may have an even longer-term effect on women's health than we previously imagined. One study found that women with an average age of sixty who had breastfeed for at least a year had significantly lower rates of cardiovascular disease and lower LDL cholesterol (Schwarz et al. 2009). Another study found lower risk of metabolic syndrome, the precursor syndrome to type 2 diabetes (Ram et al. 2008).

Effects on your baby. Skin-to-skin contact, stroking, and massage also release oxytocin in a baby's system to calm him and make him more open to your overtures. No wonder skin-to-skin contact has proved to be such a time-tested and effective tool to overcoming breastfeeding problems! As a baby enjoys skin-to-skin contact, his blood pressure decreases, his heart rate slows, and he begins to feel more open to this pleasurable, warm contact with his mother (Uvnäs-Moberg 2003). Many studies have even found that skin-to-skin contact provided pain relief to babies undergoing painful procedures (Shah, Taddio, and Rieder 2009).

Skin-to-skin contact isn't important only for premature babies. All human babies are born expecting the calming, comforting habitat of their mother's body, and every baby deserves this loving transition to life outside the womb.

When the System Breaks Down

Most of us don't think much about the role of physical touch in our lives, but its effect is much more profound than you might imagine. Right from birth, skin-to-skin contact encourages a close relationship between mother and baby and promotes breastfeeding by triggering the baby's inborn feeding behaviors, but it is more than a pleasant, nice-to-have option. Touch is vital to your baby's physical and emotional development. Of course, there are times when a mother and baby cannot be together after birth, and this loss can be made up after they are reunited. But if you have a choice, there are many reasons to do everything possible to keep your baby close from birth.

What are the downsides to the newborn of lack of touch? When full-term, healthy babies are not held, they cry more, are more stressed, and have higher blood pressure. If lack of touch becomes chronic, they are at a greater risk of feeding problems and can lose weight even if they are well fed (Uvnäs-Moberg 2003). Premature babies who do not participate in Kangaroo Care have lower survival rates (Cattaneo et al. 1998); more heartbeat and breathing difficulties (Bergman, Linley, and Fawcus 2004); more problems with oxygenation and greater stress levels (Törnhage et al. 1999); more pain experienced during procedures (Johnston et al. 2003); more sleep problems (Feldman et al. 2002); and later discharge from the hospital, greater risk of premature weaning, and relationship problems between parent and child (Charpak et al. 2001).

Long-Term Effects of Touch

In chapter 1, we described a study of full-term, healthy babies at birth in which a short separation was found to greatly affect the first breastfeeding (Righard and Alade 1990). These practices, which are still all too common, reflect a cultural insensitivity to the importance of touch and togetherness. It seems obvious that mothers and babies cannot breastfeed when they're separated and that being apart could affect breastfeeding. Yet in many hospitals and birthing facilities, little effort is made to keep mothers and babies together. Indeed, giving mother and baby time to touch and to get acquainted after birth sometimes seems more like an afterthought. That is why it is worth your while to make arrangements to stay with your baby as much as possible after birth (even if it's not standard procedure) and to arrange for your support person to act as your advocate as needed.

EFFECTS OF TOUCH ON FEEDING

Although most parents are understandably happy to cuddle with and hold their babies as a normal part of family life, some popular parenting books and programs discourage touching except at specific, prescribed times. When weighing your parenting options, it may help to know that restricted physical contact can contribute to a variety of problems. Lack of touch has been linked to feeding disorders, refusal to feed, malnutrition, and failure to thrive (Feldman et al. 2004; Polan and Ward 1994; Uvnäs-Moberg 2003). These are not just breastfeeding problems but also include problems with feeding of any kind, including bottlefeeding and the acceptance of solid foods by the older baby.

EFFECTS OF TOUCH ON ATTACHMENT AND BEHAVIOR

Touch has also been found to play a critical role in babies' emotional attachments. Research has found a correlation between healthy relationships and touch. Mothers and babies who have lots of physical contact tend to enjoy good relationships. Healthy dynamics naturally flow from lots of touch. On the other hand, relationship problems are often found in mothers and babies who spend little time touching. In one study, researchers found that togetherness and touch predicted good attachment between mothers and babies. Physical distance and separation correlated with emotional distance and attachment issues (Feldman et al. 1999). So never hesitate to pick up your baby for fear of "spoiling." That's not the way it works.

Infant carrying, even without skin-to-skin contact, has been found to help mothers be more responsive to and positive with their babies. In one study, researchers randomly assigned a group of low-income American mothers of newborns to use either soft baby carriers, which provided more contact, or infant seats, which provided less contact (Anisfeld et al. 1990). The study found the following:

- At two months of age, babies who were carried cried less and were less likely to have a daily period of crying than babies whose mothers used infant seats.

- At three months, mothers who carried their babies responded more quickly to their babies' cries than mothers in the infant-seat group.

- At thirteen months of age, infants who were carried were more securely attached to their mothers than babies whose mothers used infant seats.

The authors concluded that using a soft baby carrier helps mothers be more responsive to their infants and promotes secure attachment. These findings occurred without skin-to-skin contact.

Don't ever worry that all the time spent holding, feeding, and comforting your baby is time wasted. It is central to your baby's healthy emotional development and contributes to your lifelong good relationship.

EFFECTS OF TOUCH ON HEALTH

As we mentioned earlier in this chapter, regular touch is also critical to a baby's very survival. In his book *Touching*, anthropologist Ashley Montagu notes that, just as Dr. Bergman found in Africa, even in developed countries, touch—or lack of touch—can make the difference between life and death. Dr. Montagu reports that in the 1930s, a New York hospital decreased its infant mortality rate by providing scheduled carrying and cuddling time to the babies in its pediatric ward. Just by adding some affectionate human touch to its medical care, the hospital's infant mortality rate decreased from 30 percent to less than 10 percent. Dr. Montagu writes:

What the child requires if it is to prosper, it was found, is to be handled, and carried and caressed, and cuddled, and cooed to.... It would seem that even in the absence of a great deal else, these are the reassuringly basic experiences the infant must enjoy if it is to survive in some semblance of health (1978, 79).

So you can see that touch is far more than a nice "extra." It is vital for your baby's normal growth and development. How wonderful that science confirms what your heart is already telling you.

Touch and Your Family

Some of the previous studies and examples reflect extreme circumstances. Of course, we know (thank goodness!) that few mothers and babies will find themselves on the "little touch" to "no-touch" end of the touch spectrum. But it is instructive to know, first, that there is a spectrum and, second, which end is healthy and which end is not. That gives you a chance, as you ponder different parenting styles, to think about where on the touch spectrum you want your family to be. Once you decide, you can make your parenting choices accordingly.

When it comes to touch, research tells us that the societies and individuals on the healthy end of the spectrum are those that keep mothers and babies together and spend lots of time touching. Human biology tells us that the human baby is born expecting human milk and constant contact. That is our biological norm. Although constant togetherness and touching may not be how you were raised or how you're expecting to raise your baby, know that societies exist in which babies are never separated from their mothers. The mothers most definitely work (and work hard), but rather than leave their babies, they simply tie their babies against their bodies while they work and breast-feed whenever their babies show feeding cues.

Of course, as we know from the vast differences among the cultures of our world, human beings are nothing if not adaptable to change. But as we'll discuss in chapters 5 and 8, our own culture has made some very radical shifts in a very short period of time in the way babies are fed and cared for. The danger is that some of these changes may strain our adaptability to its limits and lead to a whole host of problems for both society and individuals (see chapter 8).

Summary

We don't often talk about biology in the same breath as parenting. But it is difficult to talk about natural laws without also discussing human norms. We realize that this perspective may not necessarily affect your choices. But it never hurts to have a broader view as you stake out your own spot on the touch spectrum. Our goal in providing you with this information is to help you find your own place as close to the healthy end of the spectrum as your circumstances and your inclinations allow.

CHAPTER 3

Getting Comfortable: The Heart of Successful Breastfeeding

> **Law 3:** *Better Feel and Flow Happen in the Comfort Zone*

The first two laws explain in large part how the dance of breastfeeding is designed to bring mother and baby close, a great example of how the physical affects the emotional. When mothers and babies first learn this dance—with each mother and baby developing their own unique variation—it is similar to learning other kinds of dances. The first time you try the movements, they feel awkward. But with practice they become easy and automatic—at times even thrilling. Mothers who grow up watching women breastfeed learn it in the most natural way. But for those of us who grew up watching babies bottlefeed, some basic knowledge can be of great help.

What Every Mother Needs to Know About Comfortable Breastfeeding

In chapter 1, we described breastfeeding as a right-brained (heart or body knowledge) activity. This is how most physical learning takes place, including things like learning to ride a bike. The same thing is true about learning to breastfeed. We've often shared this idea with mothers who have been having breastfeeding problems and are learning new ways of putting their babies to breast. Understanding that this is a learning process helped them feel less frustrated when they practiced (awkwardly at first) new strategies. It helped them relax, be patient, and keep working at it until baby's attaching to breast felt fluid and automatic.

Because we've devoted this whole chapter to this subject, we also want to emphasize that helping baby take the breast is not complicated. Although it may involve some practice at first, it quickly becomes easy. And knowing when you've got it is a snap: you know you've got it when breastfeeding is comfortable for you and your baby is thriving.

Positioning Basics

Getting comfortable involves both finding a comfortable feeding position and your nipple comfort during breastfeeding. Because both of these are so interconnected and basic to successful breastfeeding, at almost every home visit—no matter what the problem—we spend some time discussing these feeding basics. Nearly every mother and baby benefits from this. These basics include the following concepts:

- The *comfort zone* is where the nipple should be in the baby's mouth for comfortable and effective breastfeeding.

- Body positions and baby's hardwiring can be used to help the nipple reach the comfort zone.

We encourage you to visit our website (www.breastfeedingmadesimple.com), where you'll find animation that's been created to illustrate good breastfeeding dynamics in action. Why? Much of the magic is in the movements, and these can be most fully conveyed with animation. Please also keep in mind that if you're having problems, there's no substitute for a visit with a lactation consultant. In the United States, many low-income mothers have free access to breastfeeding help at their local public health departments. See the Resources section for other ways to find a lactation consultant when needed.

THE COMFORT ZONE

The comfort zone is a real place in your baby's mouth. You can find it in your own mouth by running your tongue or your finger along the roof (palate) of your mouth. As you do, you'll notice that the section of your palate nearest your front teeth is ridged or bumpy. Behind these bumps is an area that is smooth. That is your hard palate. As you continue to move back past the smooth area nearer to your throat, you'll notice that the roof of your mouth becomes soft. The comfort zone is near that area in your baby's mouth, where her palate turns from hard to soft (Jacobs et al. 2007).

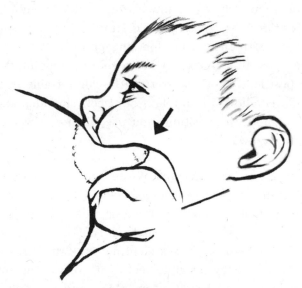

The comfort zone is an actual place in your baby's mouth near where her hard and soft palates meet. (©2005 Peter Mohrbacher, used with permission)

There are two reasons you want your nipple to reach your baby's comfort zone during breastfeeding:

1. It makes breastfeeding comfortable for you by protecting your nipple from friction and compression.

2. It gives your baby more milk, keeping her interested in and active at the breast for a longer time.

FINDING A COMFORTABLE BREASTFEEDING POSITION

Before your baby attaches to the breast, think about what feeding positions you'd like to use. When deciding, keep in mind that some breastfeeding positions may work better for you than others. Because each woman's arm length, breast size, and height are unique, a one-size-fits-all approach is not practical. What works well for your friend or neighbor may not be as comfortable for you.

A position that works for you. One reason breastfeeding has gotten the reputation of being so much work is that many mothers use feeding positions that cause muscle strain or require supporting baby's weight with their arms for long periods. We're here to help you think about this differently. From your standpoint, the best breastfeeding positions are those you can be comfortable in for up to an hour and that allow you to relax your neck, shoulder, and arm muscles. (Think about the positions you use when you watch your favorite television show.)

A position that works for your baby. We described your baby's hard-wiring in chapter 1. Now let's get more specific. Of course your baby needs to be comfortable during breastfeeding, but in some positions it is also actually easier for her to breastfeed. For example, to trigger many of the inborn feeding reflexes identified by British researcher Suzanne Colson, your baby needs to feel light pressure against her chin, torso, hips, legs, and feet (Colson, Meek, and Hawdon 2008). This can be accomplished in many positions when you are sitting up, lying on your side, or leaning back with baby's tummy down on your body. But in some of these positions, gravity can make breastfeeding harder.

HOW GRAVITY CAN HELP OR HINDER BREASTFEEDING

One amazing aspect of Dr. Colson's research was her conclusion that human babies, like hamsters and puppies, feed best on their tummies. She came to this conclusion after analyzing the effects of gravity in ninety-three videotaped breastfeeding sessions.

Sitting up straight or lying on your side. When mothers tried to put their babies to breast in these positions, gravity pulled their babies' bodies away, creating gaps between mother and baby. When this happened, many babies became frustrated and upset because their feeding triggers were missing. In the case of one upright mother, her baby's *arm-cycling reflex* was triggered, and her baby kept batting at the breast. This mother finally gave up, assuming her baby did not want to breastfeed. The pull of gravity caused other babies to arch away, making attachment difficult. In these positions, more mothers found breastfeeding to be a struggle.

Laid-back breastfeeding. When mothers used *laid-back breastfeeding* (leaning back with their babies lying tummy down on their semi-reclined bodies), the dynamics were very different. Gravity kept their babies' bodies securely against theirs so no gaps could form and feeding triggers were continuous rather than interrupted. There were far fewer breastfeeding struggles, and the mothers perceived breastfeeding more positively. This may be in part because in laid-back positions, mothers were freed from supporting their babies' weight with their arms. One mother who used a laid-back position said, "Breastfeeding is so easy. I wish more of my friends were doing it" (Colson, Meek, and Hawdon 2008, 447).

From a practical standpoint, breastfeeding in laid-back positions is a lot less work. Your body supports your baby's weight, and you don't even have to think about your baby's feeding triggers. In these positions, thanks to gravity, your baby's chin, torso, legs, and feet automatically stay in contact with your body. During the early weeks while you're in your right-brained postpartum mode, you don't have to remember ten thousand left-brained steps about how to get your baby latched on deeply. Most are taken care of for you, and you can focus on your baby instead of what you need to do next. In laid-back positions, the same feeding reflexes (such as your baby's arm-cycling reflex described above) that can get in the way in other positions make it easier for your baby to get to the breast and attach deeply so that your nipple reaches the comfort zone. And having at least one hand free makes it easier to help your baby or just to stroke and enjoy her. Laid-back breastfeeding sets the stage for the kind of intimate mother-baby moments most women dream about during pregnancy.

Your Baby Is Ready to Feed

Whatever position you use, your baby's hardwiring will respond best if her head, shoulders, and hips are in a straight line, and her chin, torso, hips, legs, and feet are pressed against your body or something else.

USING LAID-BACK BREASTFEEDING

Laid-back breastfeeding can help make the early days and weeks of breastfeeding easier while your baby is at her most uncoordinated and you're just learning the ropes. It's like the training wheels on a bicycle, which allow the rider to keep her balance as she learns the feel of riding. Conveniently, most hospitals beds are adjustable, making leaning back to breastfeed easy. The best angle of recline is one in which you're upright enough for easy eye contact with your baby but leaning far enough back so that gravity keeps your baby well-supported and tummy down on your body. When you find a comfortable angle for you both, simply lay your baby tummy down between your breasts and make your breasts accessible so she can easily make her way there.

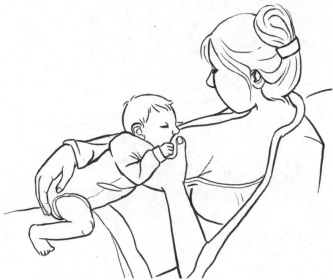

In this laid-back breastfeeding position, your baby's weight is supported by your body, making breastfeeding less work for you and easier for your baby. (©2010 Anna Mohrbacher, used with permission)

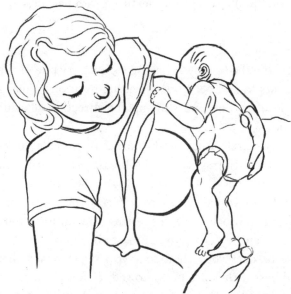

After a cesarean birth, positioning your baby across your breasts allows you to enjoy laid-back breastfeeding without pressure on your incision. (©2010 Anna Mohrbacher, used with permission)

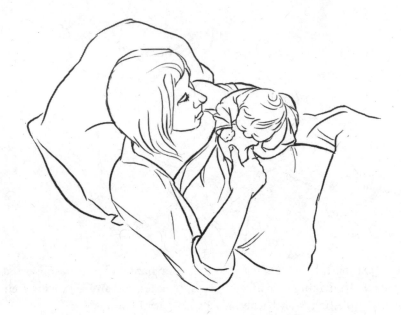

This is another laid-back breastfeeding position that can be comfortable after a cesarean birth. (©2010 Anna Mohrbacher, used with permission)

Making adjustments. If either of you is having trouble, try one of the two common adjustments to laid-back breastfeeding positions: raising or lowering your angle of recline and shifting the direction of your baby's "lie" on your body.

Because the breast is a circle, there are hundreds of possible directions from which your baby can approach the breast. She can lie on your body lengthwise with her feet by your thighs. She can lie on your body diagonally. If you've had a cesarean birth, you will probably want to avoid having your baby's weight resting on your abdomen. To accomplish this, she can lie across your breasts or approach your breast from your side or over your shoulder. Dr. Colson noted that some babies breastfed best if they are first allowed to lie in a position similar to the one they used in the womb before going to the breast (Colson 2005). (See the drawings in this chapter that illustrate some of these different lies.)

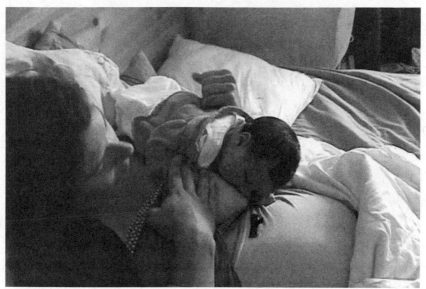

The breast is a circle, and your baby can approach it from many directions, such as this one, which could be used after a cesarean birth. (©2010 Suzanne Colson, used with permission)

As long as your baby's chin, torso, hips, legs, and feet are aligned and in contact with something (your body or, for example, a pillow along your side), her feeding reflexes will be triggered. The best laid-back positions are those in which you and your baby fit together like two pieces of a puzzle, so whichever variations of these positions you and your baby find easiest and most comfortable will be the best for you.

Your role. Because breastfeeding is part of your relationship with your baby, don't feel shy about helping her whenever it's needed. Remember, Dr. Colson's research found that mothers, too, appear to have instinctive feeding behaviors that can help trigger the right reflexes in their babies at the right time (Colson, Meek, and Hawdon 2008). Don't hesitate to interact with your baby when the spirit moves you. Breastfeeding is not just about the milk; it is also a way to get to know your baby and to express your love.

If your baby seems to be having trouble taking the breast, one way you may be able to help is by shaping the breast with your fingers (far enough back on the breast to stay out of her way) to make it easier for her to fit into her mouth. For details, see, "The sandwich analogy" later in this chapter.

The public version. You may be wondering if laid-back breastfeeding is something that is only practical in the hospital or at home. Not at all. Variations of it can also be used when you and your baby are out and about. Think about how you sit when you watch your favorite television show or when you're getting comfortable in your chair at a restaurant. Most of us don't sit bolt upright. We scoot our hips forward and lean back. Laid-back breastfeeding includes those positions, too. In most settings, some variations of laid-back breastfeeding can be used (see the drawing immediately below).

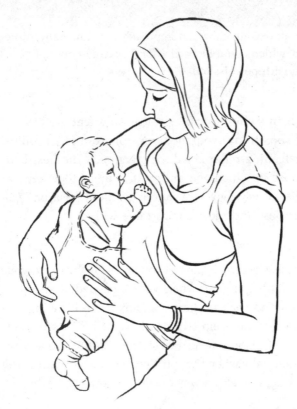

With the baby lying diagonally and the mother less reclined, this laid-back breastfeeding position could be used in a restaurant, at the movies, or anywhere. (©2010 Anna Mohrbacher, used with permission)

SITTING UP OR LYING ON YOUR SIDE

There may be some times you would rather breastfeed sitting more upright or lying on your side, and that's fine. It's always good to have choices. But in these positions, you need to take a much more active role in helping your baby attach deeply to the breast so your nipple reaches the comfort zone.

In sitting or side-lying positions, make sure your baby's whole body is facing and touching yours. A baby whose body is turned or twisted is more intent on getting comfortable than on feeding. When working against gravity with an uncoordinated newborn, providing firm touch against her shoulders helps her head, neck, and mouth feel stable, so she can feed better. Enjoy snuggling baby in close under your breasts. The closer your baby's body is to yours, the better.

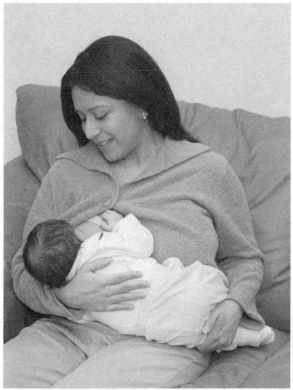

Some moms like to breastfeed sitting up, either with or without a pillow under an elbow. (©Ameda, used with permission)

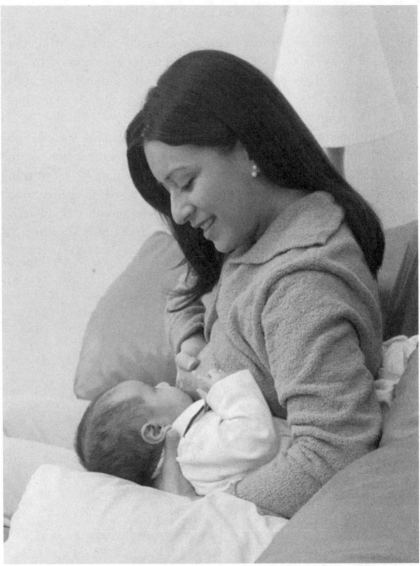

Some women like to sit up and snuggle baby along one side during feed-ings. This works especially well after a cesarean birth and for moms with large breasts. (©Ameda, used with permission)

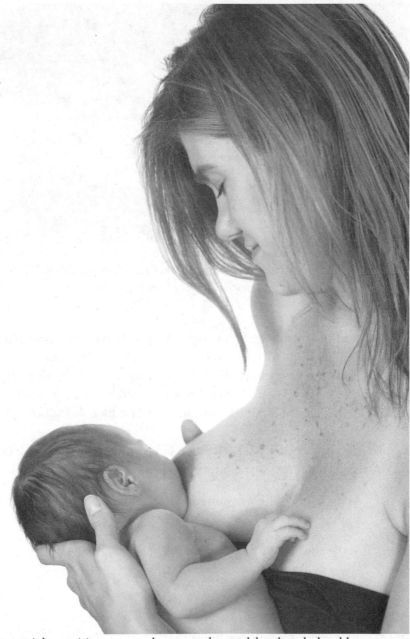

In upright positions, a newborn needs good head and shoulder support and the feel of her mother's body against hers to trigger feeding reflexes.

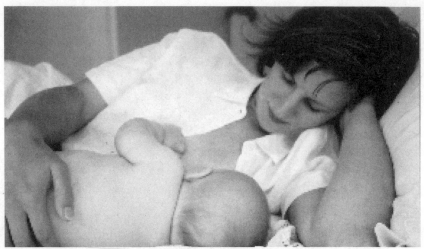

Many mothers enjoy relaxing while breastfeeding on their side. An older baby needs almost no help in taking the breast in this position. (©2005 Australian Breastfeeding Association, used with permission)

In these positions, the following basic points will help your baby most easily latch on to your breast so that your nipple reaches her comfort zone. As we mentioned earlier, it is ideal to start with a calm baby who is ready to feed. If your baby is upset, use Law 2, *Mother's body is a baby's natural habitat*, to calm her first by holding her close. Done? All right, let's start.

To achieve a comfortable, effective latch while sitting up or lying on your side, you'll follow these three steps:

1. Align baby's nose to your nipple with your baby's head tilted slightly back.

2. Make sure baby's mouth is wide open.

3. Help baby onto the breast.

Aligning baby to breast. Years ago, women were encouraged to center the nipple in the baby's mouth. We know now that this is not ideal. Experience has taught us that an off-center, or asymmetrical, latch is more comfortable than a centered latch. To achieve this, avoid lining up your baby with her mouth directly opposite the nipple. To find the comfort zone, your baby's lower jaw needs to land as far away from the nipple as possible.

Why is this? Think for a moment about how people's jaws work while they are eating. (Take special note of this the next time you have a meal.) The upper jaw stays motionless; it's the lower jaw that moves up and down. This makes the lower jaw the "working jaw" (Wiessinger 1998). Mothers find that the farther this working jaw is from the nipple when baby attaches to the breast, the more comfortable breastfeeding feels and the easier it is for the nipple to extend farther back into the baby's mouth, to the comfort zone.

If that's difficult for you to picture, imagine the opposite for a moment. If baby's lower jaw latches on right beneath the nipple, a shallow latch is inevitable. The nipple ends up just inside the baby's mouth, unable to extend back into the comfort zone.

To achieve an off-center latch, using the following body dynamics may help:

- *Nose lined up to nipple.* What this means, from a practical standpoint, is that when you are lining up your baby's body with yours (in whatever hold you choose), avoid aligning your nipple with your baby's lips. Instead, align your nipple with your baby's nose or, if you prefer, with that cute little indentation between her upper lip and nose known as the *philtrum.* When you are lined up this way, you are in perfect position for the best kind of off-center latch because the baby's lower jaw drops as she opens wide, which positions her lower jaw as far from your nipple as possible.

- *Head tilted slightly back.* Hold your baby so that her head can tilt back slightly. When your baby goes on chin first and head back, it allows you to more easily aim baby's lower jaw where you want it. Why is it helpful for a baby to have her head tilted back? As we described in chapter 1, think about how adults drink, especially when thirsty and drinking quickly. We tilt our heads back slightly to chug our drink down (try it!), because it is the easiest way to swallow. (On the other hand, try resting your chin on your chest and see how hard it is to swallow.) How you hold your baby can make swallowing easier or harder for her, too. If she is held with her shoulders pressed firmly under your breasts and her hips are pulled in tight against your body, these body dynamics make it easier for her head to naturally tilt back slightly.

- *Chin first.* If your baby's head is resting on your forearm, a "chin first" approach will probably work better if her head is closer to your wrist than your elbow. If you use a hand to support her head while she is taking the breast, try putting your palm on your baby's back and shoulders and your thumb and fingers behind her ears or, if baby is on her side, with your fingers supporting her lower cheek. Most babies do not like to have their head pushed onto the breast and will push back.

Here's a recap of the main ideas to keep in mind when the baby is getting ready to latch:

- Hold baby's body under your breasts and firmly against you (with baby's shoulders and chest pressed into your body and breast).

- Align baby's nose to your nipple.

- Allow baby's head to tilt back slightly.

- Support baby firmly behind the shoulders and back, pull her hips against you.

What to avoid. There are some aspects of your baby's hardwiring that you don't want to trigger during latch, as they can work against you. When experimenting with positions, it is wise to avoid the following:

- applying pressure to the back of your baby's head

- allowing the soles of your baby's feet to push against a hard surface

- leaving open spaces between you and your baby

When their heads are pushed, babies tend to push back. There are several reasons for this. For one, pushing on the head tilts it forward, chin to chest, making it more difficult to swallow. This may also push the baby's nose into the breast, making breathing difficult. When given the choice between eating and breathing, breathing always wins.

When the soles of a baby's feet push against a hard surface, her natural response is to push back, which can work against your efforts to relax and breastfeed. Whichever position you choose, tucking her feet against your body is one way to avoid this.

If there are large enough gaps or spaces between you and your baby, she will likely pull up her legs to fill the gap and make herself feel more secure. This pushes her body away from yours, making latching on more difficult.

A WIDE-OPEN MOUTH AND ONTO THE BREAST

Knowing that a baby latches on best with a wide-open mouth and tongue down doesn't clarify *how* to make this happen. This is another example of how understanding babies' hardwiring can make a huge difference. Many mothers who are having breastfeeding problems feel as if breastfeeding is out of control. When a mother is unclear on her baby's hardwiring, she may wrongly assume that all she has to do is put the baby near the breast and let nature take its course. But newborns need to feel specific triggers to respond this way. In laid-back positions, because gravity keeps a baby's body and chin in contact with her mother's body, this happens automatically. But when babies are fighting gravity, this contact can be easily lost, so they usually do better if they get some help from their mothers. Without this help—especially during the first few weeks—a newborn may respond to a mother's attempts at latching on by wailing and batting at her breast.

To an inexperienced mother, a baby's frustration at the breast may be a mystery. Some wrongly interpret a hungry, unhappy baby's batting at the breast as a sign that she doesn't want to breastfeed. Usually, nothing could be further from the truth. Some worry it's her way of saying that she just doesn't like breastfeeding. A mother's worst fear is that it means her baby doesn't like her!

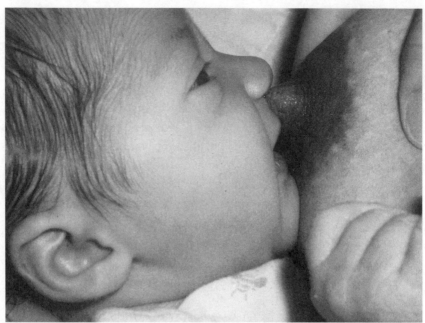

When aligning baby to breast, think "nose to nipple." (©2005 Catherine Watson Genna, BS, IBCLC, used with permission)

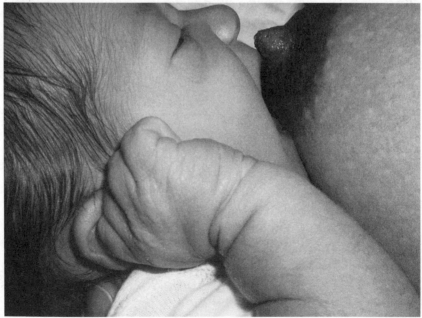

The touch of baby's chin to the breast triggers a wide open mouth. (©2005 Catherine Watson Genna, BS, IBCLC, used with permission)

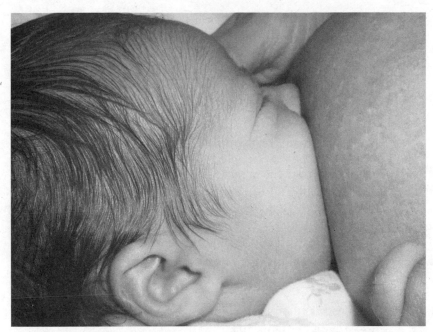

As baby tilts her head back farther and her upper gum clears the nipple, snuggle her in with a gentle push behind her shoulders so your nipple extends to the comfort zone. Note the dark area showing above baby's upper lip. (©2005 Catherine Watson Genna, BS, IBCLC, used with permission)

Use your baby's hardwiring. The good news is that understanding a baby's hardwiring puts you in the driver's seat. Once you know your baby's triggers, you can make them work for you in any position, eliminating most of the frustration and making latching on easier and calmer for both you and your baby. Learning these strategies can turn an out-of-control mother into a confident, competent breastfeeding mother.

How do you use your baby's hardwiring? As just described, in laid-back positions, the feel of the mother's body against the baby's chin, torso, hips, legs, and feet triggers the baby's inborn feeding behaviors, including positioning herself at a good angle to the breast, rooting, opening wide, and taking the breast. In laid-back positions, the touch of baby's chin against her mother causes baby to open wide. When she opens wide over the breast, gravity pulls her head down. This helps pull her farther onto the breast, making it easier for the nipple to extend into the comfort zone.

In an upright sitting position or lying on your side, this is trickier. In this case, let's assume first that you have all the right ingredients in place:

- Baby is calm and ready to feed.

- She is held near the breast, with her head, neck, and hips in a straight line and her body pulled in close enough so that there are no gaps between you and her.

- Her head is directly facing the breast, and her body is firmly pressed against yours, with her nose aligned with the nipple.

- Her head is tilted back slightly, and she is approaching the breast with her chin first.

To trigger baby's hardwiring, touch her chin with the breast. Either a light, steady touch or repeated light tapping is baby's cue to open wide and drop her tongue. Mothers are often amazed at how well this works. When a baby gets the right cues, you may see the light dawning in her eyes. Now you are speaking her language!

Lightly bring baby to the breast so that her chin is touching it. Usually, it works best to move the baby toward the breast, not the breast toward the baby. Moving the baby instead of the breast gives you more control over the process. It is less confusing this way, too, because you don't have to shift gears—from moving your breast to moving the baby—when your baby opens wide.

As we mentioned earlier, when you breastfeed sitting up, gravity makes putting your baby to breast more work for you. If you are breastfeeding in this position, you need to give your baby a gentle push from behind her shoulders as she latches on to help her take the breast deeper, especially during the first few weeks. At birth, babies have limited control over their movements. As they mature and develop, they gain body control gradually from the head down: first head and neck, then arms, and finally legs. By the time they're about four to six weeks old, babies have much more head and neck control than they did at birth and can more actively help themselves latch on deeply, even when gravity is working against them.

Before around 1980, the connection between depth of latch and breastfeeding comfort was not yet widely understood. Mothers with nipple trauma were usually told, "Just wait four to six weeks. Your nipples will toughen up, and the pain will go away." While it has become crystal clear that nipples never do "toughen up" (no matter how long you breastfeed, calluses never form on nipples like they do on a guitar player's fingers), it is indeed true that in most cases nipple pain will subside with time. Even so, a month or more is a very long time to wait when you are in pain at every feeding, and for this reason many women in earlier times stopped breastfeeding. The real reason the pain subsides after four to six weeks of breastfeeding is because, as babies develop head and neck control, no matter what position is used, they can achieve a deeper latch all by themselves, without their mother's help. Their newly gained head and neck control allows them to pull themselves farther onto the breast, which rewards them with more milk, more quickly. This deeper latch resolves their mothers' nipple pain.

We know now that even in those positions in which gravity is working against them, breastfeeding can be comfortable from birth when a mother actively helps her baby farther onto the breast. When gravity is working against you, even if all the other ingredients are in place (baby is aligned well at the breast, nose to nipple, head slightly tilted back, chin first, with wide-open mouth), your nipple will not reach the comfort zone if that last, gentle shove of the baby's shoulders is missing. Without it, baby ends up with a shallow latch. That gentle push as she latches on is a vital part of moving the nipple into the comfort zone. One word we sometimes use to describe this to mothers is "oomph."

To make latching on easier when gravity is working against you, remember the three basic concepts:

- *open* (a wide-open mouth)

- *angle* (nose to nipple; head slightly tilted back; chin first; shoulders, hips, legs, and feet pulled in close)

- *oomph* (a gentle push on baby's shoulders at latch to move the nipple into the comfort zone)

Once the baby is on with a good off-center latch, you can see some of the *areola* (the dark area around the nipple) above the baby's nose. Despite what many are told, it is not necessary or even desirable to get all of the areola into the baby's mouth. What's most important is that the baby's lower jaw takes in a big mouthful of breast. This is vital to reaching the comfort zone.

Once your baby is on the breast, look to see if her nose is blocked. If so, pull her bottom in closer. This will angle her nose away from the breast. With a great latch, your baby's chin will be in the breast, but her nose doesn't have to be. It is perfectly fine to pull your baby's bottom closer to you to give her more breathing room.

IF MORE HELP IS NEEDED, THINK "SANDWICH"

If breastfeeding is not yet comfortable, shaping the breast may make it easier to get the nipple into the comfort zone.

The sandwich analogy. To understand how to shape your breast, think about how we as adults take a bite out of a sandwich that's larger than our mouth, suggests Diane Wiessinger, MS, IBCLC, a lactation consultant in upstate New York (Wiessinger 1998). What do you do? First, you make sure you are holding the sandwich so that it is horizontal and aligned with the corners of your mouth. You don't turn the sandwich vertically, because that would make it harder to take a bite out of it.

How does this apply to latching on? No matter what position you're using, if you support your breast with your hand, be sure you are not presenting your baby with a "wrong-direction sandwich." If you squeeze your breast, be sure the mouthful of breast the baby is getting is squeezed to align with the length of her mouth. (If your finger or thumb is running parallel to your baby's upper lip, you're good to go.) For example, if you are holding your baby horizontally across your lap, the oval of your baby's mouth will be vertical, so hold your hand under your breast like a U. That way, you will be squeezing the "sandwich" in the same direction as your baby's mouth. (Be sure your fingers are out of your baby's way during latch.)

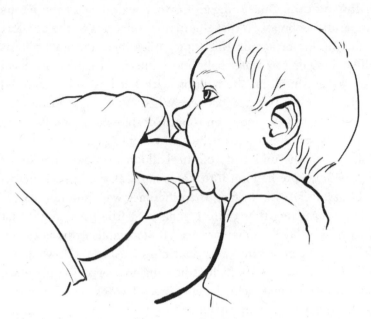

If you position your fingers parallel to baby's lips, breast shaping may make it easier for your baby to take the breast deeper. (©2010 Anna Mohrbacher, used with permission)

Another way to think about this that may help is to imagine that the finger or thumb closest to your baby's upper lip is a "mustache" for your baby. In other words, for the breast and mouth ovals to align (the right-direction sandwich), your thumb and fingers should run parallel to your baby's lips.

If sitting up or lying on your side, get into "sniff position." Think again about how you go about biting into a large sandwich. You probably hold the sandwich just above the level of your mouth and tilt your head slightly back, like a baby taking the breast. Wiessinger calls this the *sniff position*. Also, you don't usually shove the sandwich straight into your mouth. You place as much of the underside of the sandwich as you can onto your lower jaw and then "roll" the rest into your mouth. In laid-back positions, babies usually orient themselves to the breast so that they approach it at a good angle, in the sniff position.

Use a rolling motion. This rolling motion can really help a baby get the biggest mouthful of breast so that the nipple rolls back to the comfort zone. In fact, in her article on this topic, Wiessinger included photos of herself latching on to a water balloon to illustrate (really!). She used lipstick to make a mark on the balloon with her lips, which showed the different results of two approaches: When Wiessinger pushed the balloon straight into her wide-open mouth, despite her best effort, she took a relatively small amount of the balloon into her mouth. When instead she rolled the underside of the balloon first onto her lower jaw, she drew far more balloon into her mouth, as the lipstick marks showed (Wiessinger 1998). In fact, the difference was astounding!

The key to reaching the comfort zone is for the baby to get that larger mouthful of breast. One easy way to accomplish this is to roll the underside of the breast into her mouth first, just as we do when we take a bite of a large sandwich. By highlighting an everyday experience, the sandwich analogy has helped make breastfeeding more comfortable and effective for many mothers.

WITH PRACTICE, BREASTFEEDING BECOMES AUTOMATIC

After you and your baby have had some time to practice good breastfeeding dynamics, you'll be amazed at how quickly it becomes automatic. At first you may find yourself very focused on your "moves." But as time passes, you'll find you're concentrating less on what you're doing and more on how rewarding this part of your relationship with your baby is. And before you know it, you'll be one of those mothers who easily fit breastfeeding into their other activities without missing a beat. Breastfeeding will become what it was always meant to be: a normal, natural part of your life with your baby.

When the System Breaks Down

Many of the breastfeeding problems that have become so common are a direct result of poor breastfeeding dynamics and shallow latch, when the baby takes the breast but the nipple lands outside the comfort zone.

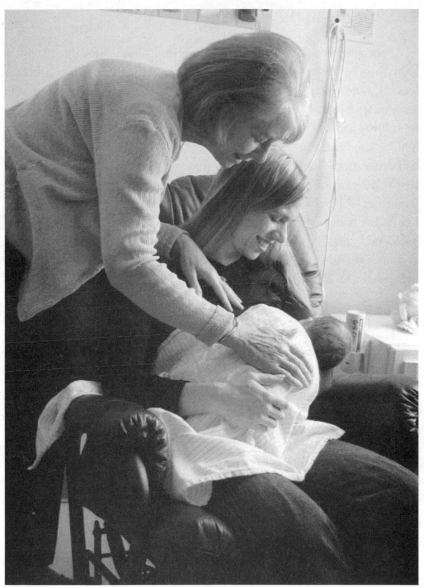

If you're having trouble getting your baby latched on comfortably, a board-certified lactation consultant can help. (©2005 Mary Jane Chase, RNC, MN, CCE, IBCLC, used with permission)

Struggles at the Breast

Poor breastfeeding dynamics sometimes make it difficult for a baby to take the breast at all. As we described earlier, when a baby's feeding reflexes are triggered but gravity is working against her, she sometimes becomes her own worst enemy at the breast by batting at it or arching away. Struggles with breastfeeding can be demoralizing to a new mother and frustrating to a newborn. When baby regularly fusses and cries at the breast, a new mom may get upset. She may be worried that this behavior means that her baby is rejecting her. She may worry about her ability to care for her baby. She may feel guilty, believing her baby's behavior is somehow her fault or that she has not given her baby good care. She may feel like a failure. Difficulty latching on is one common reason mothers give up on breastfeeding in the early weeks (Taveras et al. 2003).

If Your Nipple Doesn't Reach the Comfort Zone

A shallow latch can cause several issues that can then snowball into other problems.

NIPPLE PAIN AND TRAUMA

With a shallow latch, your baby's tongue will compress your nipple against her hard palate, causing nipple distortion and pain. Nipple distortion is hard to miss. You can see it when your nipple comes out of your baby's mouth and is oddly shaped, "smashed" looking, or pointed like a new tube of lipstick. If your baby breastfeeds with a shallow latch feeding after feeding, you may get a *compression stripe* on your nipple, which eventually leads to cracks and bleeding. Other types of trauma can occur, too, sometimes looking like a starburst or scabbing on the nipple. Shallow latch is the most common cause of nipple pain and trauma. If you have nipple pain, please refer to the section "Nipple Pain and Trauma" in chapter 10 for suggestions on what you can do. If you can't correct the problem on your own within a day or two, it is time to make an appointment to be seen by a lactation professional.

LESS MILK FOR BABY

If your baby breastfeeds with a shallow latch, this may cause pain for you, but it can also be bad for your baby because it usually means less milk at each feeding. When the nipple reaches the comfort zone, it ensures that your baby has a large mouthful of breast. The more breast tissue she has over her tongue, the more milk she can take from the breast. This triggers more active suckling for longer stretches. Taking a small mouthful of breast with a shallow latch gives baby less milk when she suckles. There are several consequences of a slow flow of milk during breastfeeding:

- A baby may lose interest quickly, falling asleep at the breast after a few minutes.

- Because the baby is not transferring milk well, she may breastfeed "all the time," taking long feedings with little time in between.

- A baby may gain weight poorly (less than 5 oz. [140 g] per week during the first three months).

Single, Double, or Triple Whammy

These problems don't always occur together. Sometimes a mother is in pain, but her baby is breastfeeding well and gaining weight fine. Sometimes a mother is comfortable, but her baby is not thriving or is breastfeeding all the time. But sometimes a mother may wind up with a double or even a triple whammy. It's possible for a mother to suffer from nipple trauma and have a baby who is gaining slowly and wants to feed all the time. But whether one or more of these are happening, improving baby's latch is the best place to start and the most likely solution.

Other Complications

Many of the common problems we'll discuss in chapter 10—from engorgement, newborn jaundice, and mastitis to low milk production—most often have their roots in nipple trauma, poor milk transfer at the breast, or both. In many cases, these issues are simply complications of latching problems. For example, the most common cause of nipple pain and trauma as well as poor transfer of milk is a shallow latch. And nipple trauma is a significant risk factor for mastitis because the broken skin on the nipple allows bacteria to enter the breast. Poor transfer of milk at the breast is a risk factor for low milk production because your rate of milk production is determined by how full or drained your breast is (see chapter 6). Understanding these dynamics is key to avoiding many common problems and to solving them when they occur.

Summary

We've devoted so much space to this subject because getting comfortable during breastfeeding, which includes getting your nipple into the comfort zone, is vital to a smooth and easy breastfeeding experience. Even if it takes some time and practice to really feel like a pro, learning good breastfeeding dynamics is well worth the effort. Someday your baby will thank you.

CHAPTER 4

The First Week of Breastfeeding

> **Law 4:** *More Breastfeeding at First Means More Milk Later*

The first few days after your baby is born is a period of tremendous change in your life. At times, you may feel overwhelmed by this huge transition and by all you need to learn. We are here to guide you through this time by giving you some specific information on what is normal and what you can expect.

During these first few days, there is one thing that will make all the difference, and that brings us to Law 4: *More breastfeeding at first means more milk later.* Law 4 is not meant to worry you. You may be concerned that following this law will make your nipples sore. Despite what you may have heard, if your nipple is in your baby's comfort zone, frequent breastfeeding doesn't cause nipple pain. Although mothers are sometimes still told to limit breastfeeding in the first days so that they won't become sore, research has found that this strategy makes no difference (de Carvalho, Robertson, and Klaus 1984). Without making sure the baby takes the breast deeply, postponing breastfeeding simply postpones sore nipples. But with your nipple in your baby's comfort zone (see chapter 3), you can breastfeed twins and even triplets and not worry about nipple damage. The best way to put breastfeeding firmly on track is to relax, respond to your baby's feeding cues, and feed frequently (which we'll describe in more detail in this chapter).

We want to give you a clear picture of what to expect in these first days. (Hint: It probably isn't what you think!) Normal breastfeeding during the first week is different from normal breastfeeding during the second week and beyond. In fact, these differences may feel tremendous. Most of what you have heard or read about normal breastfeeding will be true in your baby's second week—but not just yet.

If your baby is already older than one week while you're reading this chapter, don't skip it. It will probably give you a new perspective on your experience. And if you're having breastfeeding problems, the information in this and the following chapters provides the foundation for overcoming them. We have found that going back to basics is usually the best first step.

A Baby's Transition After Birth

To better understand why the first week is so different, let's focus first on the changes your baby faces after birth. From your baby's perspective, some startling physical changes happen at birth. Food and oxygen are no longer constantly provided through the umbilical cord. Your baby begins breathing air with his lungs. And for the first time, your baby begins taking his nourishment by mouth.

Small, Frequent Feedings

During pregnancy, few women question their ability to provide their baby with the right nourishment. After your baby is born, your body is equally well-equipped to give him just what he needs to help ease this major transition. Before birth, your baby never felt hunger; his need for food was constantly satisfied. After birth, your baby feels hunger for the first time. Using his digestive system and having intermittent (rather than continuous) feedings are new experiences. To make this transition easier, nature starts your baby off gradually, with small, frequent feedings rather than large amounts of milk right after birth.

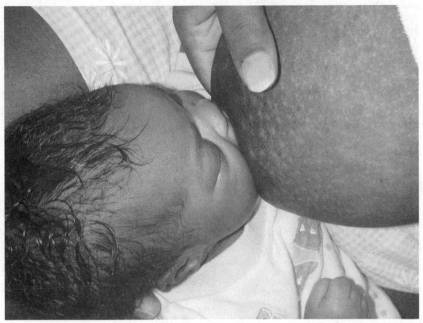

Mother's milk is all babies need during the first days after birth. (©2005 Marilyn Nolt, used with permission)

SMALL FEEDINGS

For those of us who grew up seeing babies take lots of milk by bottle right from birth, the idea of small feedings in these early days may seem strange, concerning, and, to some, even scary. In reality, these small feedings are better for your newborn than larger feedings. Why? Newborns' tiny stomachs don't stretch. Research on the size of a newborn stomach explains the experience of countless hospital nurses who have learned the hard way: when most newborns are fed 1–2 oz. (30–60 ml) by bottle during the first day of life, much of it comes right back up.

During his first day, a newborn's stomach is about the size of a large shooter marble (Seammon and Doyle 1920). At each feeding he can keep down about 1/6–1/3 oz. (5–10 ml). Not surprisingly, this is the amount of available colostrum (the early milk) that is ready and waiting for him in the breast.

Not only are newborn stomachs small, but they don't expand like adult stomachs, especially in the first day. In one 2001 study, Samuel Zangen and his colleagues found that during the first twenty-four hours of life, a newborn's stomach doesn't yet stretch the way it will later. The walls of the newborn stomach stay firm, expelling extra milk rather than stretching out to hold it. By three days of age, as the baby takes more and more of these small, frequent feedings, his stomach can expand to about the size of a ping-pong ball to hold more milk (Zangen et al. 2001). The following chart gives you a sense of how a baby's feedings increase in amount over the first month.

Baby's age	Average oz. (ml) per feeding
Three days	1 oz. (30 ml)
One week	1.5 oz. (45 ml)
Two weeks	2–2.5 oz. (60–75 ml)
One month	3–4 oz. (90–120 ml)

Would it be beneficial for you to give your newborn more milk at each feeding and try to stretch out his stomach sooner? No, this is not a case of "more is better." Why not? For one thing, small, frequent feedings set up a healthy eating pattern right from the start. Nutritionists now advise adults to eat smaller, more frequent meals, and the same is recommended for babies and children. However, many new parents are encouraged to try to give their babies as much as possible at each feeding and feed fewer times per day, which can lead to overfeeding.

A baby who is encouraged to take more per feeding may be at greater risk for obesity later in life. One study followed 653 people who had been fed formula as babies. Tracking them from birth to adulthood, the study found that gaining more weight during the first eight days of life may alter a person's metabolic programming and lead to being overweight twenty to thirty years later (Stettler et al. 2005). Other research, too, indicates that babies who are bottlefed nonhuman milks are 25 percent more likely than breastfed babies to be obese by the age of four to five years (Armstrong and Reilly 2002; Toschke et al. 2002). This may be due in part to the differences between these milks. But it may also be related to differences in feeding method. This tendency to encourage babies to "tank up" to the maximum at each feeding sets up an unhealthy eating pattern at birth that could well contribute to obesity (Li, Fein, and Grummer-Strawn 2008).

There are other reasons small feedings are better for a newborn.

Babies are born waterlogged. Imagine if you had been soaking in a bathtub for nine straight months. That's what life is like in the uterus. Although a fetus is covered with a protective layer of *vernix* (a waxy coating) to prevent his skin from becoming white and wrinkled (like ours would be if we spent that much time in the tub), all babies are born waterlogged. The last thing a brand-new baby needs is a lot of fluids. In fact, his first job after birth is to shed some of these extra fluids, which is why most babies lose a little weight at first.

Having extra fluid in the tissues at birth is a plus because it allows babies some practice time to learn to get good at taking milk from the breast before their need for fluids is great. Although in many institutions, panic begins to set in if a baby has not fed well at the breast within six to eight hours after birth, it was only about twenty-five years ago that it was standard practice in U.S. hospitals for newborns to receive nothing by mouth for the first twenty-four hours after birth. The medical professionals at the time knew that fluids were not critical during that first day of life.

This "water weight" babies are born with is the reason newborns (both breastfed and bottlefed) lose weight during the first three days. This newborn weight loss is considered within the normal range as long as it is no more than 10 percent of birth weight and is confined to the first three to four days of life (DeMarzo, Seacat, and Neifert 1991; Noel-Weiss, Courant, and Woodend 2008).

FREQUENT FEEDINGS

One of the most common questions new parents ask is when they should feed their baby. Often they are focused on the clock, because that's where much breastfeeding advice points them. However, breastfeeding has been around a lot longer than clocks, and we're going to describe a simpler way of knowing it's feeding time, one that focuses on your baby. Babies are incredibly smart, and when you tune in to your baby, you'll be amazed at how much he can tell you. Doing this is also a great way to become a more sensitive parent, which will serve you well over your child's lifetime.

Responding to early feeding cues. Although many parenting books describe how a new parent eventually learns to tell the difference between a "hungry cry" and a "tired cry," babies should ideally be fed before they are crying at all. In its statement on breastfeeding, the American Academy of Pediatrics (the professional organization that informs pediatricians on what's good practice) states that crying is considered "a late indicator of hunger" and parents are encouraged to feed their babies before they get to this point. Ideally, they say, babies should be fed when they are showing the early feeding cues we described in chapter 1 (AAP 2005b).

What are these early feeding cues? Although your newborn cannot talk, he is telling you he is ready to breastfeed when you see these cues:

- rooting (turning his head from side to side with a wide-open mouth)

- putting his hand to his mouth

As we discussed earlier, a baby who is hungry but not yet frantic is going to better respond to his hardwiring and more easily take the breast in the best possible way. In contrast, a baby who is upset and crying has a more difficult time settling down, latching on, and feeding well.

From an adult perspective, less crying means less stress for you. Your baby's crying is meant to have a profound emotional effect on you. Nature made us this way so that we would respond promptly to our baby's needs. This is a survival mechanism, and it is not healthy to try to override it. Your responsiveness to your baby is an important part of becoming a sensitive parent. This doesn't mean that you need to be constantly on tenterhooks awaiting your baby's cry or that you should beat yourself up if you're unable to catch your baby's cues before he cries. It does mean that training yourself to tune out your baby's crying (his most fundamental way of communicating) increases your emotional distance, which is a less-than-ideal beginning to your relationship.

Less crying also means less stress from a baby's standpoint. There are few people today who believe the old idea that crying is good for a baby's lungs. (Some people counter this old chestnut with, "Just like bleeding is good for a baby's veins.") In fact, research has shown that crying is not only stressful for you, but is stressful for your baby, too. Crying raises levels of *cortisol*, a physical indicator of stress, in a baby's body. So although there will probably be times your baby will cry in spite of your best efforts, avoiding crying when possible is good for everyone. The most important emotional lesson of a baby's first year is learning to trust that his needs will be met. And there is no more fundamental need than being fed when hungry.

Rooming in at the hospital. Of course, being able to respond to your baby's feeding cues assumes that you and your baby are together. This may or may not be true depending on where you give birth. For many years, babies were routinely removed to a central nursery at night and during visiting hours. Today, in many places, there is more appreciation of mothers' and babies' need to be together to establish breastfeeding. However, it is never wise to assume anything. If you have not yet given birth, it is well worth a phone call to find out what your hospital's "rooming-in" practices are. There are still some institutions in which separation is routine. Even so, it may be possible to make special arrangements so that you and your baby can stay together and have a better start.

Why frequent feedings on the first day are important. One study done in Japan demonstrated the importance of frequent feedings after birth (Yamauchi and Yamanouchi 1990). The researchers found that more breastfeedings in the first twenty-four hours correlated strongly to less weight loss, more stools, less jaundice, and greater milk intake on days two, three, and five in its 140 babies (the researchers did not provide information about day four). We'll describe this study in more detail in the last section of this chapter ("When the System Breaks Down").

Normal Breastfeeding Patterns

Now let's cut to the chase. What can you expect during these early days? Part of helping your baby transition from the constant feeding in the womb to the intermittent feeding on the outside will involve lots of breastfeeding during these early days. As described earlier, your baby is born with a small stomach. He gets small amounts of colostrum, the early milk, at each feeding. These small amounts digest quickly. For many babies, this translates to some periods of very frequent and sometimes nonstop breastfeeding.

As we'll discuss in more detail in chapter 5, newborns do not typically breastfeed at regular intervals. While it is true that babies tend to feed eight to twelve times every twenty-four hours, the usual laws of mathematics simply don't apply here. During the first six weeks or so, your baby probably won't feed on any kind of regular schedule. Most new babies tend to bunch their feedings together at certain times and go longer between feedings at other times. If you're lucky, these longer stretches (up to four to five hours is fine) will be at night—but don't get your hopes up at first (see the next section, "Baby Confuses Day and Night"). Those longer stretches will probably be during the day. So while it is a good idea to keep track of the number of feedings every twenty-four hours (see the section "Keep a Written Log" on this), ignore the intervals between feedings for now and don't expect any consistency in the intervals between feedings until your baby is older. There may be times of the day or night when your baby breastfeeds every half hour or every hour. That's all just part of normal breastfeeding in the early days and weeks.

If your baby is like most newborns, during these first days there will be times when he is breastfeeding almost constantly, possibly for hours at a stretch, going back and forth from breast to breast. When you try to put him down, he will begin to fuss and show feeding cues. Some people use the word "squirrelly" to describe how babies act during this time. This is not unusual, and if it happens to you, it's not a sign that baby isn't getting enough or that breastfeeding is not working. It is a sign that your baby is doing his job well in the days before your milk increases.

Oh, and one more thing: during these first few days, these long feeding stretches are most often at night.

BABY CONFUSES DAY AND NIGHT

One recent study confirmed what many new mothers suspect—that most babies are born with their days and nights mixed up. Babies tend to sleep more during the day and breastfeed more at night. In a study designed to help determine what is normal, Australian nurse midwife Stephanie Benson observed the feeding patterns of thirty-seven healthy, exclusively breastfeeding mothers and babies during their first sixty hours after an unmedicated birth. She found these babies fed least often from 3 a.m. to 9 a.m., while their frequency of feeding increased during the day. These babies fed most often from 9 p.m. to 3 a.m. (Benson 2001).

There are some theories about why babies are born this way. One holds that during pregnancy, babies are lulled to sleep during the day, when their mothers are active and moving, and are alert at night, when their mothers lie still. But no one knows for sure why babies mix up night and day. We only know that it is typical for newborns.

Here in the United States, most mothers arrive home from the hospital on the second day. If this is true for you, this means that during your first night home, your usual sleep time will probably coincide with your baby's peak desire to breastfeed.

COPING WITH NIGHT FEEDINGS

What's the best way to handle your baby's feeding frenzy during the wee hours? It's most important that you understand that it's normal and that "this too shall pass." If you have mastered laid-back breastfeeding (see chapter 3) and breastfeeding lying down, you're all set. **Note:** For more information on breastfeeding lying down, including safe-sleep strategies, see chapter 5.

Hopefully, your partner or support person can give you some extra help that first night home so you can sleep and breastfeed without worrying about waking up with sore nipples.

A good strategy is to get into bed at your usual time (or earlier, if you want), arrange yourself and your baby in bed so that it is easiest for the baby to take the breast or to pull baby onto the breast whenever needed. If you're lying on your side, be sure you have whatever pillows you need under your head and behind your back so that you can relax all your muscles and go right back to sleep while baby breastfeeds. (But don't put pillows around your baby, as this could be dangerous.) As your baby wakes you for feedings, help him to breast or have your partner or support person help you get your baby well latched on. If lying on your side, wedge a rolled-up small towel or baby blanket behind your baby's back (but not his head) so he has the support he needs to stay on the breast. Be sure his head is free to angle back so that he can latch on chin first. He will come off the breast when he's done, and you can hold him against your body and roll over to the other side when he wants the other breast. Or you can lean over toward him to offer the upper breast (see the photo in chapter 5 on page 124), whichever works best. While laid-back breastfeeding positions usually come easily to mother and baby, most mothers find that it takes some practice to get good at breastfeeding lying down, especially during the early weeks when the baby is most uncoordinated. But it is well worth the effort to find comfortable positions in which you can get your rest, even if you need a second person's help at first (see chapter 5 for more specifics, safety tips, and lots of photos). Once you have it mastered, there is no muss, no fuss, and no one has to lose much sleep.

When breastfeeding in bed at night, some mothers worry about how and when to change baby's diapers and what to do about burping. Breastfed babies tend to take in much less air than babies who feed by bottle, so they may or may not need to be burped at all. (With just a little experience, you'll quickly get a sense of your own baby's needs.) During these first few days, a baby is unlikely to be gulping down lots of milk anyway, as it comes in small amounts. So if your baby falls back asleep without burping, let him be. He will wake and fuss if he needs to burp. Regarding diapers, it is practical to have a changing station set up next to your bed. But there is no need to change diapers during your normal sleeping hours unless the baby has a bowel movement. And during these first few days, this is a great job to assign your partner or support person.

Another important way to get the rest you need and to recover from birth is to make a pledge to sleep when baby sleeps. This may be at times when you would normally be awake and getting things done. Keep in mind that you just had a baby and your body and mind will need time to adjust. Be sure to accept all offers of help. This is the time to hunker down and get on your baby's rhythm.

If your baby's internal clock says that midnight to 3 a.m. is party time, there are some tried-and-true strategies you can use to help baby learn that nighttime is for sleeping. (For more on these strategies as well as getting attuned to baby's rhythm, see chapter 5.)

Breastfeeding Basics

Now let's focus on the basics you need to make breastfeeding work.

One Breast or Two?

A common question mothers ask is whether they should give both breasts at each feeding or if they should give just one. The answer is "neither." Ideally, your baby will make this decision. When a baby is healthy and breastfeeding normally, he is fully capable of determining when it's time to switch breasts. After all, he's the only one who knows how much milk he's had and if he's ready to go to the other side.

FINISH THE FIRST BREAST FIRST

Not too long ago, the most common advice given to breastfeeding mothers was to breastfeed for ten to fifteen minutes on the first breast, take the baby off, and then keep him on the other breast for as long as he liked. This strategy worked well for many mothers and babies, but there were some for whom it didn't work.

DISADVANTAGES OF BREASTFEEDING BY THE CLOCK

For the lactation professionals trying to help these mothers, the problem was mysterious. The moms obviously produced a lot of milk, but their babies were not gaining weight well. The babies were also colicky, gassy, and had green, frothy stools. They were not happy campers! Eventually, when the cause of their problem was discovered, we gained a new insight into an aspect of breastfeeding that had not been widely understood.

The issue was that these mothers had been following the standard advice to switch their babies to the second breast after ten to fifteen minutes. Michael Woolridge, Ph.D., a British physiologist, and Chloe Fisher, a British midwife, were the researchers who solved this mystery. In 1988, they described to the world in the medical journal *Lancet* how this way of managing breastfeeding had caused the problem. Fat, they explained, sticks to the milk ducts in the breast. This means that when the breasts are full, the first milk that is released is low fat. As the breast is drained and more milk is pushed toward the nipple, fat is dislodged from the ducts into the milk, increasing its fat content. By switching breasts too soon, these babies had gotten mostly low-fat milk on the first breast. Then they were switched to the other breast where they also received mostly low-fat milk, having filled their bellies before reaching the higher-fat milk. This overload of low-fat milk rushed through their digestive systems, causing the gas, the colic, and the low weight gain (Woolridge and Fisher 1988).

Now we understand that the fat content of milk gradually changes during each feeding and that in some unusual cases breastfeeding "by the clock" can prevent babies from getting to the fattier milk on either breast. The first milk a baby gets (sometimes called *foremilk*) is lower in fat (in some cases like the 1 percent cow's milk we might buy from the store). As baby continues to feed, the milk increases in fat (more like 2 percent milk). As the baby continues to drain the breast, the fat content increases until it is as fatty as whole milk, then half-and-half, then cream (sometimes called *hindmilk*).

Fortunately, once it was understood that the babies who were having these problems were receiving mostly low-fat milk, the solution was simple: leave the baby on the first breast until he finishes it. When the baby receives both the low-fat and the fattier milk, milk will no longer rush through his system. The higher fat content of the fatty milk causes it to linger longer in the intestines, preventing the gas and colic and boosting baby's weight gain. More-recent research from Australia has found that for most babies, milk-fat content balances out no matter what feeding pattern is used (Kent et al. 2006), but the British mothers studied had very overabundant milk production.

The Easy Way Is to Follow Your Baby's Cues

In many ways, this finish-the-first-breast-first approach makes breastfeeding blissfully simple. You don't need a clock. You don't need to worry about your milk's fat content. (Later in this chapter, we'll explain in more detail how your baby's stools tell you he's had enough of the fatty milk.) Just leave your baby on the first breast until he either pops off on his own and seems finished on that side or falls asleep and comes off. Then change his diaper to see if this extra stimulation makes him interested in taking the other side. (Don't plan to change him right before a feeding, when he's frantic. No doubt by the time he finishes the first breast, it will be good to change him anyway.) If he wakes and is interested in taking the other breast, go ahead and give it. If not, that's fine, too. Once your milk increases on the third or fourth day, most babies take one breast at some feedings and both breasts at others.

This strategy relies on your baby's ability to tell you what he needs. As with us adults, some babies are fast eaters and some are slow eaters. So a clock will never tell you when your baby is done. (How would you feel if, in the middle of your meal, someone pulled your plate away?) Only your baby knows for sure when the flow on one breast has slowed down to the point where he is ready for the other side. Only he knows when he's had the right amount of milk for that feeding. And only your baby knows when he's had just the right mix of the thinner foremilk and the fattier hindmilk. You have no way of knowing, and thankfully, this is one thing you don't need to know. Your baby gets to decide— which is the first step toward healthy eating habits.

Every Baby Is Different

Be suspicious of any parenting books that recommend the same feeding pattern for all mothers and babies, because individual differences can profoundly affect these dynamics. Many mothers with a large breast storage capacity (see chapter 6) find that their babies always take one breast at a feeding. Mothers with smaller or more average milk storage often find that their babies always want both breasts. There are no hard-and-fast rules, because mothers and babies are individuals and these individual differences are responsible for the natural variations in babies' feeding patterns. (We'll describe this in more detail in chapter 6.)

During these first days, as we discussed, the amount of milk available to your baby tends to be small to match the size of his stomach, and your baby may want both breasts at every feeding. In fact, in these early days, your baby may want both breasts several times at each feeding. Don't hesitate to give each breast more than once if your baby seems to want it. Let your baby be your guide.

How to Know When Breastfeeding Is Going Well

The first time a mother breastfeeds, she often worries about whether it's going normally. For those used to bottles, it may seem unsettling that our breasts don't have markers allowing us to see how much milk goes into baby at each feeding. But fortunately, there are other ways to know that a breastfed baby is getting enough milk. Once you can identify the signs, you can relax and enjoy your baby.

Birth to Day Four

The following sections focus on the important areas that prompt most women's questions as well as some easy-to-identify signs that can tell you how breastfeeding is going.

YOUR BREASTS

After birth, your breasts will feel soft until the milk increases on the third or fourth day. Sometimes this is incorrectly referred to as the milk *coming in.* This description is misleading because it implies that prior to this, you have no milk. Because of this misunderstanding, many newborns have been given unnecessary supplements of formula. The truth is that you have had milk in your breasts during much of your pregnancy. As we described in the introduction, the amount of colostrum, the early milk, your baby receives provides exactly what your baby needs nutritionally and has components needed for the normal functioning of your baby's digestive and immune systems.

During these early days, few women feel much breast fullness. This is helpful for your baby, because it gives him some practice at taking milk from a soft breast before any firmness occurs. With this early practice, your baby will find it easier to handle any changes in breast texture that occur as your milk production increases.

BABY'S WET DIAPERS

You may have heard that new babies should have five or six wet disposable diapers every twenty-four hours and at least three to four yellow stools. This will be true later but not yet. Misunderstandings about this are another common reason babies are given formula unnecessarily.

We described earlier in this chapter why, during these first few days, the amount of colostrum, the early milk, is small: Your baby has a small stomach and can't handle more. (It would most likely just come back up because the newborn's stomach can't stretch.) He is also born waterlogged and doesn't need more fluids. In fact, during this time, he needs to shed fluids to reach a healthier balance.

Because the amount of colostrum baby gets is small at first, the number of wet diapers will also be small until your milk increases on the third or fourth day. Here's what you can expect:

- day one: one wet diaper

- day two: two wet diapers

- day three: three wet diapers

- day four: four wet diapers

As you can see, as your baby takes his small, frequent feedings, your milk production gradually increases. By the end of the first week, the volume of your baby's output will likely be ten times greater than the day he was born.

BABY'S STOOLS

The first stools your baby passes are called *meconium*. These are black, tarry, and sticky and are not made from your milk; they were in your baby's intestines before birth. As you will see later in this chapter (in "When the System Breaks Down"), passing the meconium quickly is important in preventing exaggerated newborn jaundice. Fortunately, colostrum has a laxative effect, which causes meconium to pass very naturally during normal breastfeeding.

When your baby is breastfeeding well, your baby's stools should begin to change from black to greenish (called *transitional stools*) by day three or four. If a baby is still passing black meconium stools after day four, it's time to take your baby for a weight check. **Note:** If he has lost more than 10 percent of birth weight, find skilled breastfeeding help to evaluate what needs adjusting (see Resources) because your baby is at risk for underfeeding.

By day five, your baby's stool should turn yellow (Nommsen-Rivers et al. 2008; Shrago, Reifsnider, and Insel 2006). In a nutshell, if breastfeeding is going normally, at a minimum, you should see the following:

- day one: one stool (black)

- day two: two stools (black)

- day three: three stools (black or greenish)

- day four: three to four stools (greenish or yellowish)

If you're keeping track of your baby's stools, which we recommend, keep in mind that in order to count, a baby's stool should be the size of a U.S. quarter (about 2.5 cm) or larger. Smaller stools are fine (and your baby will no doubt have stools of different sizes); they just don't count.

If your baby's stool turns to greenish or yellow ahead of schedule, that's great. It just means that breastfeeding is going especially well.

Often new parents are surprised by the appearance of a breastfed baby's normal stools. They look nothing like adult stools and, fortunately, they smell nothing like them either. Rather than being formed, the normal stools of a breastfed baby are very loose. Some compare them to the consistency of split pea soup, with lots of liquid and some curds. They may look seedy or completely watery. Both are normal. They may also vary in color. Once the meconium is completely passed, normal stools can be anything from tan to yellow to green.

Due to the healthy effect of human milk on a baby's gut, when babies are exclusively breastfed, their stools have a mild, inoffensive scent. Once a baby receives any other food, his gut flora changes and so does the fragrance of his stools.

BABY'S WEIGHT

As we said before, newborns (both breastfed and bottlefed) typically lose weight during the first few days after birth while they shed their excess fluids. In a 1991 study, researcher Sandra DeMarzo and her colleagues found that when mothers received good breastfeeding guidance and support, babies lost no more than 7 percent of their birth weight during these first three to four days (DeMarzo, Seacat, and Neifert 1991). A weight loss of up to 10 percent is considered in the normal range, but if your baby has lost 7–10 percent of birth weight, it may be time to take a closer look at breastfeeding to make sure baby is feeding well; some adjustments may be needed. **Note: Babies should reach their low weight by four days of age. If a baby is still losing weight after four days, seek skilled breastfeeding help immediately.**

Even if a baby's diaper output is within the normal range, a weight check is suggested. The American Academy of Pediatrics recommends that every newborn be seen by his doctor at three to five days of age (AAP 2005b). If a baby has fewer-than-expected wet diapers and stools, it's important to know that the baby scales available at most baby stores are not accurate enough to rely on during this time. Neither is the strategy that occurs first to many new parents, which is to get on the bathroom scale alone, then with the baby, and subtract the first weight from the second. Instead, a doctor's or lactation consultant's scale should be used to check the baby's weight and the baby should be naked (no diaper) when weighed. Most scales used by board-certified lactation consultants are accurate to either 0.1 oz. (2 g) or 0.35 oz. (10 g), and some doctors provide free weight checks for their patients.

BABY'S FEEDING PATTERN

Normal feeding patterns can vary in the first few days of life. When breastfeeding is unrestricted, some babies breastfeed for several hours at a stretch, switching back and forth many times from breast to breast, then sleeping for several hours, and repeating this pattern until the milk increases on day three or four. This is one of the reasons that having help is often recommended during this time. Having someone on hand to take care of all the other household responsibilities while mother just sleeps and breastfeeds makes this process much easier. Some babies breastfeed for short periods, ten to fifteen minutes, but feed every thirty to forty minutes around the clock. If your baby follows either of these first two common feeding patterns, take heart! This is an intense period, but it doesn't last long. And if you follow your baby's lead and breastfeed like crazy at first, you will most likely be one of the lucky ones whose milk increases quickly and whose baby is soon satisfied for longer stretches.

Some babies, particularly those whose mothers received medication during labor or whose labors were very long and difficult, may seem uninterested or sleepy during these early days. However, they need their mother's milk as much as other babies. If your baby is sleeping so much that he doesn't wake for at least eight feedings in twenty-four hours or he falls asleep within the first few minutes of breastfeeding, you may need to help him. Disregard the oft-repeated adage, "Never wake a sleeping baby." Although you may not need to wake him completely, putting baby to breast is exactly the right thing to do. British researcher Suzanne Colson, whose work we described in chapters 1 and 3, found that newborns—even late preterm newborns—can actually feed very effectively while in a light sleep (Colson, DeRooy, and Hawdon 2003). If your baby is swaddled, unwrap him. Make sure he's not overdressed or too warm, which can make him sleepy. Hold him against you in laid-back positions. When you see signs he's in a light sleep (like eyes moving under eyelids, mouth movements, any sort of movement), try helping him to the breast. He may surprise you by taking it.

The most important number to track in these early days is the number of feedings. The goal is to make sure a baby breastfeeds well at least eight to twelve times per twenty-four hours.

PASSING LOTS OF GAS IS NORMAL

During these first few days, when a baby is using his digestive system to process food for the first time, it is normal to pass lots of gas. As the baby takes colostrum and its laxative effect begins to work, his digestive system will start to function normally. Gassiness is part of this normal early functioning and is not related to your diet. (See chapter 9 for more on diet and breastfeeding.)

Days Four to Seven

Days four to seven mark the next phase of early breastfeeding. Many aspects of breastfeeding begin to change as your milk increases.

YOUR BREASTS

There is a range of what's normal when milk production increases. When babies breastfeed long and often during the early days, some women never feel particularly full, even after their milk has increased. Knowing this can be a great motivator to follow the natural laws. More typical, though, is some feeling of breast fullness while milk production increases. Mothers usually find during this time that their breasts become larger, heavier, and perhaps tender. Keep in mind that more is happening in the breasts than just making extra milk. Extra blood is also drawn to the breasts to aid in increased milk production, causing some of the swelling you may experience. An IV during labor can also cause excess tissue fluid to be retained, causing further swelling.

If breastfeeding does not go well in the early days and the breasts are not well drained of milk, women are at risk for breast engorgement. If this happens, the breasts become very firm and full. They may also be hard and/or hot. Engorgement can be extremely uncomfortable and is well worth avoiding if possible. If your breasts become engorged, see chapter 10 for suggestions about what you can do. The good news is that if engorgement is treated, it usually only lasts for twelve to forty-eight hours.

If a baby is breastfeeding well, normal breast fullness usually only lasts about two to three weeks. Once the hormones of childbirth have settled down and milk production becomes well established, the breasts begin to feel normal and feelings of fullness subside. Some women mistakenly believe that because their breasts no longer feel full, their milk has disappeared. This is definitely not the case. The heaviness and fullness of the early weeks is not a permanent part of breastfeeding.

BABY'S WET DIAPERS

Once the milk has increased on the third or fourth day, baby's wet diaper count increases dramatically. The baby who had one, two, or three wet diapers per twenty-four-hour day suddenly begins wetting five or six diapers. Several events coincide to make this possible. Your baby's stomach begins to stretch out so that he can take 1–1.5 oz. (30–45 ml) at feedings, and mother's milk production increases to that level. At one week, the shooter marble–sized stomach of the newborn has stretched to almost the size of a chicken egg. More milk made and drunk is reflected in more wet diapers—typically five to six in a twenty-four-hour day.

BABY'S STOOLS

There is also a dramatic change in a baby's stools during this time. In the previous section ("Baby's Stools" under "Birth to Day Four"), we described the change in color and amount that occurs from birth to day four. By now, the black meconium that baby was born with should be completely out of his system. The stools of a four-to-seven-day-old baby are made entirely from the milk he has been drinking since birth.

A baby's stools are a very important indicator of his effectiveness at the breast and a mother's milk production. This is because the stools come from the fatty hindmilk we described in the section above "Finish the First Breast First." In order to get to this fattier milk, your baby needs to drink well enough and long enough to drain the breast well. If a baby spends time at the breast but doesn't take the milk effectively (what some lactation consultants call "being at the bar, but not drinking"), he may get the low-fat milk and have plenty of wet diapers but get very little of the fatty milk. This becomes obvious when the stools don't come or there are fewer of them than expected.

If a baby is not producing stools, this is a serious matter. It may mean that he is not breastfeeding effectively. It may mean that his mother is not producing milk in sufficient amounts. Or it may mean both. When a baby is not feeding effectively and draining the breast, his mother's milk production will not be well stimulated. **Note: If a newborn five days of age or older has fewer than the minimum three to four breastfed stools at least the size of a U.S. quarter (2.5 cm) in a twenty-four-hour period, it is time to take a closer look. And the first thing to look at is the baby's weight.**

BABY'S WEIGHT

A baby's weight is the "acid test" of how breastfeeding is going. How do you know if your baby's lack of stools is a cause for concern or just an unusual but normal variation? That's easy: you check your baby's weight. A baby should reach his lowest weight on the third or fourth day.

As we said earlier, the American Academy of Pediatrics now recommends that all babies be seen by their health professional within a few days of discharge from the hospital (AAP 2005b). This makes it possible to catch problem situations early enough that babies are not at risk.

An average weight gain for a fully breastfed baby is about 7–8 oz. (200–230 g) per week, starting from the low weight at day three or four, with boys gaining faster than girls (WHO 2006). Many breastfed babies gain more than this. A minimal acceptable weight gain is 5 oz. (140 g) per week (ILCA 2005). If your baby is gaining less than that, it is time to seek skilled breastfeeding help.

BABY'S FEEDING PATTERN

You'll probably notice that as your milk increases, not only does your baby's diaper output increase, but you'll probably hear your baby swallowing more during breastfeeding and he will seem content for longer stretches afterward. This is all part and parcel of having more milk. However, as we'll discuss in detail in chapter 5, it is still too early for most babies to fall into a regular feeding pattern. As mentioned, at one week, your baby's stomach is still just a little smaller than the size of a chicken egg. (An adult's stomach is the size of a softball!) Because his stomach is small and he is still very immature, it's normal for a baby to bunch his feedings together (or *cluster nurse*) during some parts of the day. One four-to-five-hour sleep stretch is also considered normal, and there is no reason to wake your baby during this longer stretch, as long as he is getting at least eight to twelve feedings per twenty-four hours. This cluster feeding is a normal feeding pattern for most breastfed babies during the first six weeks or so, until a baby's stomach grows larger and, with practice, they are able to take milk more efficiently. We'll describe this in more detail in chapter 5.

Regarding length of feeding, on average (and not all babies are average), most newborns breastfeed actively (with enough jaw movement to make their ears wiggle!) for a total of about twenty to forty minutes at each feeding. Some pauses during feedings are normal. As we discussed earlier, ideally a baby should be allowed to finish the first breast first, get a diaper change (during your normal waking hours) to stimulate interest, and then be offered the other breast. Usually, babies take one breast at some feedings and both breasts at some feedings. If your baby's feeding length is not average, it is easy to tell if this is a normal variation or a cause for concern: get your baby's weight checked. If your baby is gaining well, then you can stop worrying. When a baby is thriving, all is well.

KEEP A WRITTEN LOG

During the first week or two after birth, while you and your baby are learning to breastfeed, we recommend that you keep track of two things: number of breastfeedings (at least ten minutes total of wide jaw movements per breastfeeding) and number of stools of at least the size of a U.S. quarter (2.5 cm).

It is actually better to keep this simple, as the more complicated your log, the more difficult it is to interpret. You don't really need to know how many minutes your baby spends on each breast or any of the other small details. A simple log like the following will better help you keep your eye on the bottom line:

1. Get a blank piece of paper of any size.

2. Draw a line down the middle.

3. Decide when you'd like to start your twenty-four-hour day (now is fine) and write the date and time at the top of the paper.

4. Mark one column heading as "# breastfeedings."

5. Mark the other column heading as "# stools."

6. Make a tally mark for every breastfeeding with at least ten minutes of active suckling (one breast is fine).

7. Make a tally mark for every stool the size of a U.S. quarter (2.5 cm) or larger (start tracking this after your baby's stools have turned yellow, greenish, or tan).

8. Count your totals at the end of each twenty-four-hour period.

Counting your totals is the most important step. The number of feedings should be eight or more. The number of yellowish stools the size of a quarter or larger should be three to four or more. If your baby is not waking to feed at least eight times or is not feeding long enough, help him to the breast in laid-back positions when he's in a light sleep (and see "Sleepy Baby" in chapter 10 for other suggestions). If after day four, the number of stools is less than three to four, adjust your latch (see chapter 3), use the breast compression technique (described in "Sleepy Baby" in chapter 10), and make arrangements with your baby's health care provider to bring your baby in for a weight check.

After day four, a baby who is having fewer yellow stools but is gaining weight normally is fine, meaning this should be considered a normal variation for this child, though it is unusual.

Exclusively breastfed newborns do not become constipated. *Constipation*, or hard, dry stools, is a common digestive side effect of infant formula. Because most health professionals are not trained in breastfeeding norms, many mothers of exclusively breastfed babies are erroneously told when their baby is not producing stools, he is constipated and should be given a suppository. **Note: A fully breastfed baby younger than six weeks not passing enough stools is a red flag for underfeeding, and his weight should be checked as soon as possible.** Giving a suppository only delays getting appropriate help, prolongs the problem, and puts your baby (and breastfeeding) at risk.

COUNT WET DIAPERS?

Some suggest also keeping track of wet diapers, but this is really not necessary. As we explained before, the first milk your baby gets at the breast is the thinner, watery, lower-fat milk. The fattier hind-milk comes after, and it is the fattier milk that creates the stools and increases the baby's weight. So if your baby has enough stools, you know that he has already received plenty of fluids earlier in the feeding. You can cross that off your worry list.

We like to simplify in this way because counting wet diapers can be very difficult, especially when an ultra-absorbent disposable diaper is used. The average amount of urine a newborn voids is only about a tablespoon (15 ml). Between the small amount of urine and the absorbency of the diaper, it is really hard to tell when one of these diapers is wet.

When the System Breaks Down

The frequent feedings of normal breastfeeding may sound overwhelming, but if your baby breastfeeds well and often in the early days—at least eight to twelve feedings every twenty-four hours—you'll avoid common problems that you definitely don't need.

When breastfeeding is delayed, restricted, or unnecessarily supplemented, or when baby feeds ineffectively, possible side effects include the following:

- painful breast engorgement in mother

- a delay in increased milk production and excessive weight loss in baby

- exaggerated newborn jaundice

Engorgement

When the amount of milk you produce increases dramatically on the third or fourth day after birth, some breast fullness is common. When a mother is engorged, her breasts become very full, very firm, sometimes hard, and sometimes hot. Severe engorgement can also be painful. In the past, engorgement was considered normal for breastfeeding mothers. We know now that it is not.

Mothers often mistakenly believe that engorgement is caused by the increase in milk production. But that is only part of the picture. Engorgement is caused by the congestion of many fluids in the breast, including extra milk, blood, and tissue fluid retention aggravated by IVs used during labor. The good news is that engorgement is usually short-lived, provided that a baby is able to latch on and drain milk well from the breast. The more often and well the milk is drained, the more quickly the extra blood and other fluids can drain away, which both prevents and treats engorgement. (For more, see "Engorgement" in chapter 10.)

Delay in Milk Increase

Lack of frequent feedings in the early days may also delay the onset of more plentiful milk. A study of 140 newborns in Japan sheds light on the role of frequent feedings in increasing milk production faster (Yamauchi and Yamanouchi 1990). This study compared babies who breastfed less than seven times during their first twenty-four hours of life to babies who breastfed between seven and eleven times during the same period. The babies who breastfed more frequently took 86 percent more milk on their second day, 54 percent more milk on their third day, and 86 percent more milk on their fifth day. Not surprisingly, the babies who breastfed more than seven times during their first twenty-four hours also lost less weight and regained their birth weight faster.

Exaggerated Newborn Jaundice

If you don't yet know about newborn jaundice, now is a good time to learn. All mammals are jaundiced to some degree after birth. You know a baby is jaundiced by the yellowish tinge to his skin. A little jaundice is normal and is even considered by some to be beneficial. But if the levels get too high, newborn jaundice can be dangerous. High jaundice levels may mean frequent blood tests for your baby, repeated trips to the doctor, rental of expensive equipment, and even rehospitalization—all best avoided. Although it is very rare, babies have even died from the effects of very severe jaundice.

When babies don't breastfeed frequently in the first few days, they are more likely to have exaggerated newborn jaundice. That is because *bilirubin*, the substance responsible for jaundice, builds up without frequent feeding. Excess bilirubin leaves a baby's system via his stools; colostrum, the early milk, has a laxative effect, thereby speeding this process. The study cited in the previous section found a strong correlation between fewer breastfeedings in the first twenty-four hours and newborn jaundice on day six (Yamauchi and Yamanouchi 1990). The more a baby breastfeeds, the more stools he passes and the lower his bilirubin level.

These numbers may help you see this relationship more clearly. In this study, exaggerated jaundice on day six was confirmed in

- 28 percent of the babies who breastfed zero to two times in the first twenty-four hours;

- 24.5 percent of the babies who breastfed three to four times;

- 15 percent of the babies who breastfed five to six times;

- 12 percent of the babies who breastfed seven to eight times;

- 0 percent of the babies who breastfed nine to eleven times.

In other words, during their first twenty-four hours, the more times the babies breastfed, the fewer the cases of exaggerated jaundice that developed on day six. Not surprisingly, more breastfeedings on the first day of life also correlated strongly with the passage of more stools. And the benefits of frequent breastfeeding extend beyond the first day.

If your baby is jaundiced, see "Exaggerated Newborn Jaundice" in chapter 10 for more information on what you can do. The American Academy of Pediatrics has published treatment guidelines for newborn jaundice (AAP 2004), but not all doctors know about them. We also have these guidelines on our website (www.breastfeedingmadesimple .com). Print these out and talk with your baby's doctor about them.

Summary

Frequent breastfeeding during your baby's first days can prevent many of the problems many people assume are the normal consequences of breastfeeding in the early weeks. Knowing what you can expect from your baby and yourself in this first week can help you recognize when things are going well or when it's time to seek support from a knowledgeable lactation specialist.

CHAPTER 5

How Your Baby Sets Your Milk Production

> **Law 5:** *Every Breastfeeding Couple Has Its Own Rhythm*

All of us approach breastfeeding with expectations about what it will be like, but reality often proves to be far different. To make it work, you need to find and follow your baby's natural feeding rhythm. What does that mean? That's the main focus of this chapter.

The Adjustment Period

In chapter 4, we discussed how the size of a newborn's stomach affects her feeding pattern during the first week. Moving forward in time, after the first week, the baby's stomach size is still a major player. Other factors include her ability to take milk faster and the natural ebb and flow of your milk production over the course of a day.

For most parents, the first forty days are especially challenging. No wonder it's called "the adjustment period." No matter how a baby is fed, most new parents find that caring for a newborn is surprisingly intense and sleep is at a premium. When you begin breastfeeding, it may feel uncoordinated. As the weeks go by, you and your baby will feel more coordinated in more feeding positions and breastfeeding gets easier and faster. You and your baby begin to settle into a new "normal" in your lives. During this intense time of constant feedings and diaper changes, keep in mind that after these first forty days usually comes what we like to call "the reward period."

One physician we know has a standard pep talk he gives new parents who are worried that breastfeeding is too much work. He draws a graph of the postpartum period, with weeks along the bottom and amount of work along the side. Then he draws two lines, one representing breastfeeding and one representing bottlefeeding. His breastfeeding line starts higher, and he acknowledges that at first, breastfeeding can feel like more work than bottlefeeding. But at around five weeks the lines cross. Once mother and baby have become practiced at

The "Work" of Breastfeeding

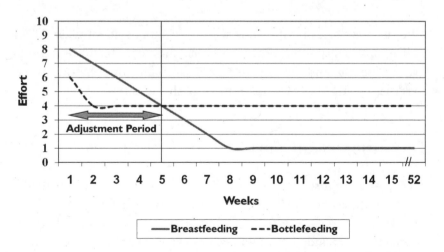

At first, breastfeeding may take more time and effort than bottlefeeding, but within about five weeks—as babies get faster at feedings—bottlefeeding takes more time. Ultimately, breastfeeding is a huge time-saver. (Concept: Peter Rosi, MD; Graphics: Nancy Wight, MD, IBCLC)

breastfeeding, it suddenly becomes far less work than bottlefeeding, which requires shopping, preparation, washing, and wide-awake night-time feedings. After the lines diverge, bottlefeeding stays at the same higher level, while the work of breastfeeding drops.

His main point is that getting breastfeeding established initially is indeed a time investment. But it is an investment that pays back many times over. Breastfeeding saves innumerable hours (and much money) over the long run.

During these first forty days, you can make the journey from "adjustment" to "reward" easier or harder, according to the choices you make. These choices most definitely affect breastfeeding, but there is much more to it than that. They also lay the foundation for your relationship with your child. How you respond to your baby in the first months of her life can affect both her physical and mental health. Breastfeeding is so much more than food. To give you some ideas about strategies that can help, let's see how this time is viewed in other cultures.

The First Forty Days

In many parts of the world, the first forty days after a baby is born are considered to be a time distinct from everyday life. Mothers are pampered and cared for. They are fed and bathed. They are encouraged to breastfeed and focus primarily on the new relationship with their baby.

Those of us who have had babies in the United States are painfully aware of how different it is here, especially the pressure to "get back to normal" as quickly as possible. Within the span of a generation, longer hospital stays and an assumed recuperation period after childbirth have given way to new mothers at the shopping mall right after hospital discharge and women returning to work within their baby's first month. As we will see, this may be one reason why the incidence of "baby blues" and postpartum depression is so high.

Rushing back to what used to be normal is not the best way to handle this vulnerable time. The postpartum period has not always been this way in the United States and is handled much differently in other parts of the world.

HOW OTHER CULTURES SEE IT

Suzanne Arms, author of *Immaculate Deception* (Bantam, 1977) and a longtime advocate of holistic birth and parenting, once asked "Is ours not a strange culture that focuses so much attention on childbirth—virtually all of it based on anxiety and fear—and so little on the crucial time after birth, when patterns are established that will affect the individual and the family for decades?" (personal communication). Many of us in industrialized countries often act as if we have nothing to learn from developing nations, yet many of these traditional cultures do something extraordinarily right in the way they care for new mothers. After studying postpartum practices in a wide number of cultures, anthropologists Gwen Stern and Larry Kruckman noted in their classic 1983 cross-cultural review that postpartum depression (including the milder form known as the "baby blues") was almost unheard of in many countries. In contrast, in developed countries like the United States, 50–85 percent of new mothers had the baby blues, and 15-25 percent experienced the more severe postpartum depression (Kendall-Tackett 2010a).

WHAT MAKES THE DIFFERENCE?

These anthropologists found that all the cultures with a low incidence of baby blues and postpartum depression had several things in common. Not surprisingly, these key factors involved the support and care new mothers receive. Here's what these cultures did to help ease new mothers into motherhood:

- *The postpartum period is distinct.* In almost all the societies studied, the postpartum period is seen as a time distinct or different from normal life. Something that we remind our American audiences about is that this used to be the norm in colonial America, where it was referred to as the *lying-in period.* This is also a time when experienced mothers help new mothers learn the fine art of mothering.

- *New mothers rest and are cared for in seclusion.* During the postpartum period, new mothers are recognized as especially vulnerable, which is why social seclusion is widely practiced. While they rest, they are expected to restrict their normal activities and to stay relatively separate from others, except for midwives and female relatives. This rest and seclusion helps promote frequent breastfeeding and the mother's recovery following birth. Postpartum is a time for the mother to rest, regain strength, and learn to care for her baby.

- *Mothers are relieved of household duties.* For seclusion and mandated rest to be practical, mothers' normal workload must be taken on by others. In these cultures, women are provided with someone to take care of older children and take over their household duties. As in the colonial period in the United States, women in other cultures often stay in their parents' homes during this time, where help is more available.

- *A woman's new status is publicly recognized.* In these cultures, much personal attention is given to the mother; this is often described as "mothering the mother." In some places, the new status of the mother is recognized through social rituals, such as bathing, washing of hair, massage, binding of the abdomen, and other types of personal care (Stern and Kruckman 1983).

The following describes a postpartum ritual performed by the Chagga of Uganda:

Three months after the birth of her child, the Chagga woman's head is shaved and crowned with a bead tiara, she is robed in an ancient skin garment worked with beads, a staff such as the elders carry is put in her hand, and she emerges from her hut for her first public appearance with her baby. Proceeding slowly towards the market, they are greeted with songs such as are sung to warriors returning from battle. She and her baby have survived the weeks of danger. The child is no longer vulnerable, but a baby who has learned what love means, has smiled its first smiles, and is now ready to learn about the bright, loud world outside (Dunham 1992, 148).

THE REVERSE CINDERELLA

In contrast, the new mother in the United States today receives greater concern and support before her baby is born. While a woman is pregnant, people offer to help her carry things, open doors for her, and ask how she is feeling. Friends give her a baby shower, where she receives emotional support and gifts for her baby. There are prenatal classes and prenatal checkups, and many people question her about the details of her daily experience.

Increased focus on the baby. After she has her baby, however, focus on the mother vanishes. A new mother is usually discharged from the hospital twenty-four to forty-eight hours after a vaginal birth, or two to four days after a cesarean birth. She may or may not have anyone to help her at home—chances are no one at the hospital has even asked. Her mate will probably return to work within the week, and she is left alone to make sure she has enough to eat, to teach herself to breast-feed, and to recuperate from birth. The people who gave her attention during her pregnancy are usually no longer there, and the people who do come to visit are often more interested in the baby than in the mother. There is the unspoken understanding that she is not to bother her medical caregivers unless there is a medical reason.

Is it any wonder that many women find the postpartum period extremely stressful? In one book written for new mothers, *What to Expect the First Year*, authors Arlene Eisenberg, Sandee Hathaway, and Heidi Murkoff describe this transition as "the reverse Cinderella—the pregnant princess has become the postpartum peasant" with a "wave of the obstetrician's wand" (Eisenberg, Murkoff, and Hathaway 1989, 546).

Options for postpartum support. Chances are it will be many years before care will be provided for new mothers through the U.S. health care system. But in the meantime, a grassroots movement has arisen to meet the needs of postpartum women. Those who take on this role are called *doulas*, from the Greek word for "servant." A doula provides practical and emotional help to women before, during, and after birth and can be a friend, family member, or a woman's partner. In some places, professional postpartum doula services are available. If you don't have someone to provide hands-on, practical help after birth, and if you can afford it, we strongly recommend hiring a postpartum doula. (See our Resources section and website for ways to find doula services in your area.)

We need to learn from other cultures and begin to change the way we think about the kind of care new mothers need. Care should ideally continue throughout the first forty days. The "I-can-tough-it-out" attitude our culture encourages in new mothers will serve neither you nor your baby well. A new mother needs help to recover from childbirth, to make the emotional transition to motherhood, and to breastfeed her baby.

Breastfeeding Norms

These first forty days are vital to both your adjustment to motherhood and to successful breastfeeding. One important task of the postpartum period is learning your baby's breastfeeding rhythm, which is our next topic. In this section, we walk you through what you can expect.

Your Milk Production

In chapter 4, we described how, with frequent feedings, your milk production increases dramatically during your baby's first week of life. Let's look now at how your baby sets your milk production during the weeks that follow.

THE AMAZING FIRST MONTH

The first month is a critical time for your milk production. After you give birth, your body is primed and ready to make milk. The hormones of pregnancy have prepared your breasts by stimulating the growth of your milk-producing glands. When your baby is born, the separation of the placenta from the uterus triggers the hormonal chain of events that causes your milk to increase on the third or fourth day. During the first month your baby's breastfeeding stimulates even more breast growth and development.

The first week. As we discussed in chapter 4, by the end of your baby's first week of frequent breastfeeding, your milk production will have increased ten-fold—from a total of about 1 oz. (30 ml) per day on day one to about 10–12 oz. (300–360 ml) per day by days five to seven.

During this same time, your baby's stomach expands from about the size of a large shooter marble to about the size of a chicken egg. Your baby can now comfortably take about 1–1.5 oz. (30–45 ml) of milk at a feeding. As your baby grows, her stomach keeps growing and so does your milk production.

The second and third weeks. With frequent feedings, your milk production continues to build. Now your baby can hold about 2–3 oz. (60–90 ml) at a feeding and takes about 20–25 oz. (600–750 ml) of milk per day.

This is also a time when babies often increase the number and length of breastfeedings. This is not only because she's hungrier than she was; this also serves to increase your milk production to meet her growing needs. When this happens, you'll know your baby is doing exactly what she is supposed to do. Experienced mothers have observed that these periods of longer, more frequent feedings (sometimes called *growth spurts*) often seem to happen at around two to three weeks, six weeks, and three months.

The fourth week. Your baby is now taking about 3–4 oz. (90–120 ml) per feeding, and her intake has increased to about 25–35 oz. (750–1,050 ml) per day. Amazingly, at around one month you are producing just about as much milk per day as your baby will ever need. (For more on this, see chapter 6.)

In control of your breastfeeding destiny. There are many good reasons to exclusively breastfeed during the first forty days if at all possible. In addition to all the health issues, exclusive breastfeeding makes it easier to meet your long-term goals. When your baby sets your milk production at "full," you're in the driver's seat.

With full milk production at one month, you can make whatever choices you like in the months ahead. If you want to breastfeed your baby for the recommended minimum of one year, you are set to go. You can always change your mind, but in the meantime, you have everything you need to meet any long-term breastfeeding goal you set.

Increasing milk production is usually more difficult later. Although mothers have done it, it is usually more difficult to increase milk production after one month. By then you are past the point when the hormones of childbirth are working in your favor. Women who increase their milk production later find that it usually takes two to three times longer than if they had worked on it within the first two weeks. And in some unusual cases, no matter how hard they try, they just can't budge it.

We don't yet completely understand why this is so. There is a theory that during the first week or two after birth, frequent breast-feeding (or pumping) activates a certain number of prolactin receptors in your breast that determine your maximum milk production for this baby. If a mother does not activate enough prolactin receptors during that time, the theory goes, she may not establish what it takes to reach full production (de Carvalho et al. 1983).

Knowing whether you have full milk production is easy. If your baby is exclusively breastfed and is gaining 5 oz. (140 g) per week or more, you're just fine.

THE DAILY EBB AND FLOW

There is more to understanding milk production than knowing how much milk you make and how much your baby takes every twenty-four hours. A breast is not like a spigot, with the milk at the same level day and night. Your milk production has its own natural ebb and flow, which affects your baby's feeding pattern.

Morning abundance. Morning is the time when milk production is usually at its highest. Mothers who express or pump their milk find that they tend to get more milk in the morning than they do later in the day. Mothers who exclusively breastfeed often report that their babies go longer between feedings during the morning hours than in the evening. Why is that?

When scientists measured the hormonal levels of breastfeeding women, they found that prolactin, the hormone long thought to be related to milk production, is at its highest level in the middle of the night. That may be one factor, but there are no doubt others. As babies turn their days and nights around to be more in tune with the rest of the family, they breastfeed less at night, which means more milk accumulates in a mother's breasts by morning.

Evening low ebb. In the evening, milk production is at its lowest ebb, and to get the milk they need, babies need to feed more often. Experienced breastfeeding mothers know that the baby who was happily full for hours between feedings in the morning is often the same baby who wants to feed every hour—or even every half hour—during the evening. Mothers who express their milk also often report that, as day turns to evening, the amount of milk they can pump decreases in amount. This is a completely normal pattern and does not mean that your milk production is low.

Sometimes called "the witching hour" in the United States or the "cactus hour" in Australia, this feeding frenzy often happens just about the time a mother's thoughts turn to getting dinner on the table. In some cases, these frequent feedings may continue all evening.

The bottom line. What's important about this for your baby is not the ebb and flow; it's the total amount of milk she gets over a twenty-four-hour period. Experienced mothers know how to plan for these predictable evening feeding frenzies. They prepare their evening meal in the morning to avoid the frustration of trying to keep their fussy baby happy while assembling dinner.

For you, the important thing to keep in mind is that "this too shall pass." As you'll see in chapter 6, these evening breastfeeding marathons are usually confined to the adjustment period of the first forty days. Once your baby is bigger, her stomach has grown, and she learns to get more milk more quickly, your breastfeeding rhythm will change, usually becoming more predictable.

Why a Rhythm vs. a Schedule?

If a mother's breasts gave the same amount of milk day and night, and if all mothers produced milk in exactly the same way, a feeding schedule could work well. But that's not reality. This is why being flexible—especially while your baby is setting your milk production—is important. The ebb and flow of milk production is one of the natural variations that affect a baby's feeding rhythm. We will discuss the individual differences among mothers in more detail in chapter 6. Suffice it to say now that the amount of milk a mother can comfortably hold in her breasts (which varies considerably among mothers) has a major effect on how often her baby needs to feed to grow and gain weight, as well as to keep up her milk production. This variation also affects a baby's feeding rhythm.

Because of our culture's focus on getting things done, many new parents feel pressured to quickly get their babies on a feeding schedule. Some strident schedule proponents assert (without *any* scientific basis) that schedules, or "parent-directed feedings," somehow promote self-discipline in a child. Some even try to make a connection between feeding schedules and God's design for mankind, even though clocks are a relatively recent man-made invention.

Yet for all the reasons we've discussed, this is the time when a schedule is least appropriate. As British baby expert Penelope Leach writes:

> Over time the behaviors that drive parents crazy change, but they do so when, and only when, the infant's physiology has matured to the point that she is a settled baby rather than a newborn. That may take three weeks or it may take six, but the we-must-do-something approach is likely to prolong the process as well as make it more painful both for parents and infants (cited in Mohrbacher 1993, 41).

There are risks in taking charge and ignoring your baby's natural feeding rhythm (which we'll discuss in the section "When the System Breaks Down," below), but one major drawback to schedules is that you have no way of knowing if your baby has gotten the right amount of milk at a particular feeding. When your baby is healthy and breastfeeding is going normally, your baby is the only one who knows if she's getting what she needs. When we parents attempt to manipulate this equation, we're in danger of throwing the whole system out of whack. (For more on the feeding schedule and its roots in "scientific mothering," see chapter 8.)

To gain a broader perspective on feeding rhythms, a quick biology lesson is in order. With so many ways of raising children, we may wonder if a biological human norm really exists when it comes to infant feeding. But many hints can be found in our biology. So stay tuned and see how we compare to other mammals.

THE IMMATURITY OF THE HUMAN NEWBORN

Some of the differences between us and other mammals are obvious at birth. Human babies are much less mature when they are born than most other mammal newborns. Why? With a larger brain and smaller pelvis, a baby's head is in danger of growing larger than a mother's pelvic region can accommodate, so a human baby is born before her brain matures completely and her head gets too big to fit through a pelvis. Most other mammals are born at about 80 percent of adult brain growth. But humans are born at less than 50 percent, with most brain growth occurring after birth. Human babies must finish their gestation outside the womb, and the ingredients unique to human milk play a key role in this.

WHAT KIND OF MAMMAL ARE WE?

To understand this, we again draw from the work of Nils Bergman, an MD from South Africa who has also studied animal biology and behavior. Dr. Bergman describes four distinct types of mammals and how the composition of their milk is related to how they care for their young (Bergman 2001a; Kirsten, Bergman, Hann 2001). The differences in the milk they produce and in the maturity of their newborns tell us which type of care is right for each. Let's see where the human infant belongs.

Cache mammals. The deer and rabbit, like other cache mammals, are mature at birth. Their mothers hide their young in a safe place and return to them every twelve hours or even less often. Consistent with this behavior, the milk of cache animals is high in protein and fat. It sustains the young animals for a long time, because the babies are fed infrequently. If it didn't, crying out from hunger before their mothers returned would make them vulnerable to predators.

Follow mammals. The giraffe and cow are follow mammals and, like others of this group, are also mature at birth and can follow their mothers wherever they go. Since the baby can be near the mother and feed often throughout the day, the milk of a follow mammal is lower in protein and fat than that of a cache mammal.

Nest mammals. The dog and cat are examples of nest mammals and are less mature than cache or follow mammals at birth. They need the nest for warmth, and they remain with other young from the litter. The mother returns to feed her young every two to four hours or so. The milk of nest mammals has less protein and fat than cache mammals. But it has more than the milk of follow mammals, who feed more frequently.

Carry mammals. This group includes apes as well as marsupials (such as the kangaroo). The carry mammals are the most immature at birth, needing the warmth of the mother's body, and are carried constantly. Their milk has low levels of fat and protein, and they are fed often and around the clock.

What type of mammals are humans? We can figure that out by looking at the content of human milk. Human milk is among the *lowest* in fat and protein content of all mammalian milks, meaning that humans are also carry mammals. Because of human infants' immaturity at birth, they need to feed often and are meant to be carried and held.

IT'S NOT NICE TO FOOL MOTHER NATURE

As we'll describe in chapter 8, many of our cultural beliefs run directly counter to our biological norms. Human evolution is all about adaptation to change. But in three or four short generations, Western industrialized cultures have attempted to make some very radical changes in how we parent our young. For example, we have made these changes over the last three generations:

- from "carry" infant care to "cache" infant care

- from continuous feeding to "nest" care (every two to four hours)

- from species-specific food to nonhuman milks (from a "follow" species—the cow)

These kinds of radical changes can strain many mothers and babies beyond the limits of their adaptability. Dr. Bergman questions if violating these basic biological norms may have led to the major increases in stress-related illnesses and other problems, ranging from ADHD to child neglect (Bergman 2001a). A growing body of scientific literature indicates that these recently adopted Western parenting styles may not really be such a good idea.

When Breastfeeding Is Going Well

There is no doubt that by breastfeeding your baby, you are taking a significant step in the right direction. To make breastfeeding effective and enjoyable, it's important to get into the proper rhythm.

YOUR BREASTS

As we said in chapter 4, if a baby is breastfeeding well, breast fullness between feedings usually lasts only about two or three weeks. Once the hormones of childbirth have settled down and milk production becomes well established, your breasts begin to feel normal and feelings of fullness between feedings subside. At this point, you will only feel full if you have an unusually large milk production, miss a feeding or two, or go very long between feedings. Some women mistakenly believe that because their breasts no longer feel full between feedings that their milk has disappeared. This is definitely not the case. As we said in chapter 4, the heaviness and fullness of the early weeks is not a permanent part of breastfeeding.

BABY'S DIAPERS

Just as they were at the end of the first week, a baby's stools are a very important indicator of how effective she is at the breast and the state of your milk production. As we explained in chapter 4, the stools are produced from the fat in the milk. If a baby spends time at the breast but does not take the milk effectively, she may get the low-fat milk and have plenty of wet diapers but may lack the calories she needs. This quickly becomes obvious when there are fewer stools than expected.

If a baby is not producing the expected number of stools, this is a serious matter. It may mean that she is not breastfeeding effectively, you are not producing enough milk, or both. **Note: If, during the first forty days, your exclusively breastfed baby has fewer than the minimum three to four stools the size of a U.S. quarter (2.5 cm) or larger in a twenty-four-hour period, it is time to take a closer look.** And the first thing to look at is the baby's weight.

BABY'S WEIGHT

Just as in the first week, a baby's weight is the "acid test" of how breastfeeding is going. How do you know if your baby's fewer-than-normal stools are a cause for concern or just an unusual but normal variation? That's easy. You check your baby's weight. After a baby stops losing weight on the third or fourth day, an average weight gain for a fully breastfed baby is about 7 or 8 oz. (200 or 230 g) per week, with boys gaining faster than girls (WHO 2006). Many breastfed babies gain more than this. A minimal acceptable weight gain is 5 oz. (140 g) per week (ILCA 2005). If your baby is gaining less than that, it is time to seek skilled breastfeeding help to see what needs adjusting.

YOUR BABY'S UNIQUE BREASTFEEDING RHYTHM

You and your baby are individuals. If babies are allowed to find their natural feeding rhythm, you'll probably find that your neighbor's baby does not feed exactly like your baby, even when both are thriving. The neighbor's baby may breastfeed more times or fewer times. She may feed for a longer or shorter period. You'll also probably notice differences in the feeding rhythms of your first, second, and subsequent babies.

Expect cluster nursing. Because your baby's stomach is still small and she's still learning how to take milk well from the breast, it's normal for babies to bunch their feedings together (or cluster nurse) during some parts of the day. This concept of cluster nursing is the closest thing we've heard to the way most newborns actually breastfeed. As we described earlier, the most common time for babies to cluster their feedings is in the evenings. When she is clustering, your baby may want to feed every hour, every half hour, or even continuously for a time.

Your baby will probably not cluster feed for long. After the first forty days, most babies fall into more regular feeding patterns. Regular, longer stretches between feedings happen as a baby's stomach grows larger and can hold more milk. Feedings also tend to get shorter as a baby gets more practiced at breastfeeding and she can drain the breast faster and more efficiently. Babies outgrow the need to cluster nurse when they can hold more milk and learn to drink more quickly.

Understanding normal feeding patterns is critical because the most common reason given for giving up on breastfeeding is worries about milk production. We believe this is largely due to the general ignorance of normal breastfeeding patterns. New parents are often told that newborns breastfeed eight to twelve times per day (a true statement), and they do the math and assume that their babies will want to breastfeed every two to three hours (not normally true). Unfortunately, some health care providers will also offer the same misguided advice. When their babies begin cluster nursing, parents mistakenly assume that something has gone horribly wrong with breastfeeding. Understanding Law 5 (*Every breastfeeding couple has its own rhythm*) allows you to relax, enjoy your baby, and go with the flow (no pun intended!).

Feeding length and one breast or two. At the beginning of these forty days, newborns tend to breastfeed actively for a total, on average, of about twenty to forty minutes. As we discussed in chapter 4, the ideal at each feeding is for the baby to finish the first breast first, then change her diaper to stimulate her interest (during normal waking hours), and then offer her the other breast. Most babies take one breast at some feedings and both breasts at some feedings. As your baby gets older and more practiced, feedings tend to shorten. So the baby who was breastfeeding for thirty minutes may drop to fifteen or twenty minutes.

In the normal range vs. average. It's important to understand that while some feeding patterns are "average," there's not necessarily anything wrong if a baby does not follow these patterns. We've met babies who were doing fine and who fed faster, fed fewer times, and passed fewer stools. We'll never forget the mother of a three-month-old very chunky baby who, when we asked her how many times per day her baby was breastfeeding answered, "five." This mother and baby were obviously not average, and yet they were also obviously in the normal range because this baby was thriving.

We've also met babies at the other end of the spectrum, who fed longer, fed more, and passed huge numbers of stools and were doing fine too. There is a whole spectrum of what's normal for babies, and "average" is just in the middle of the bell curve.

But if your baby is well outside average, don't just assume everything is fine. Have your baby's weight gain checked. (As we said earlier, a bathroom scale is not good enough. You need to take your baby to the doctor's or health care provider's office.) If she is gaining at least 5 oz. (140 g) a week, you can relax and consider your baby's feeding behavior in the normal range as opposed to average. If your baby is thriving, everything else you're doing is fine.

Normal sleep patterns. One four-to-five hour sleep stretch is considered normal during this time. There is no reason to wake your baby during this longer stretch, as long as she is breastfeeding at least eight to twelve times per twenty-four hours or is gaining well.

Coping Strategies for the First Forty Days

For those of us more familiar with bottlefeeding, breastfeeding norms can seem odd and sometimes overwhelming. We offer the following suggestions to help make this adjustment period easier for you and your family.

KNOW WHAT TO EXPECT

Don't underestimate the importance of having good information. Knowing that cluster feeding is normal has saved many breastfeeding relationships. And don't expect a doctor, nurse, or other health care provider to necessarily know breastfeeding norms. Most health professionals receive little or no breastfeeding education. This means that it's in your and your baby's best interest for you to learn about breastfeeding. Then, when you are given conflicting advice, you will have a solid basis on which to judge it.

WAYS TO GET YOUR REST

This is not the time to be Superwoman. Make your rest a priority. You're worth it!

Accept all offers of help. Take a page from the book of mothers in traditional cultures and keep the focus on you and your baby by gratefully accepting all help.

Sleep when baby sleeps. In these first forty days, your baby may have her longest sleep stretch during your usual waking hours, and you can take advantage of that to catch up on your rest. Make a pledge right now that you will sleep when your baby sleeps. If your baby is sleeping, stop worrying about writing thank-you notes, shopping, cleaning, or making meals. Get on your baby's rhythm. Remember what other cultures do, and even if no one else around you is doing it, start a new trend by allowing yourself to be pampered.

Adjust your night owl's body clock. If your baby is like most, she was born with her body clock telling her that "night time is the right time." Once your milk has increased and breastfeeding is going well, you can use some tried-and-true strategies to help her switch from night to day. But count on the fact that it will probably take a few weeks to make a significant change.

The key is to make your usual sleeping hours as boring as possible for your baby. Keep the lights low. To see well enough to help your baby attach deeply, use a nightlight or turn on a closet light and crack the door. Keep it quiet. Don't turn on the TV or radio. Change your baby's diaper only when she has passed a stool; wait until morning to change wet diapers. Keep the night hours as unstimulating as possible. Before you know it, your baby will realize that days are where the action is.

BREASTFEEDING LYING DOWN

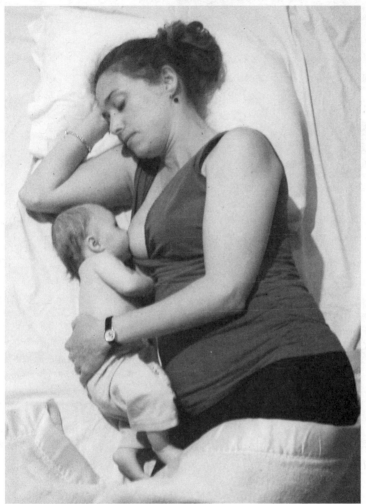

To keep baby pulled in close, either use a hand or wedge a rolled towel or baby blanket behind baby, leaving her head free to tilt back as needed. (©2010 Mary Jane Chase, RNC, MN, CCE, IBCLC, used with permission)

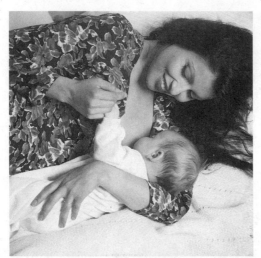

This mother feels more comfortable with her lower arm around her baby.
(©2005 Medela, Inc., used with permission of Medela, Inc., McHenry, IL)

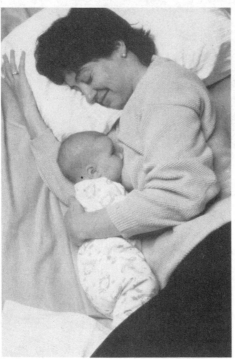

This mother feeds her baby from the upper breast without having to roll
over. (©2005 Pat Bull, RN, used with permission)

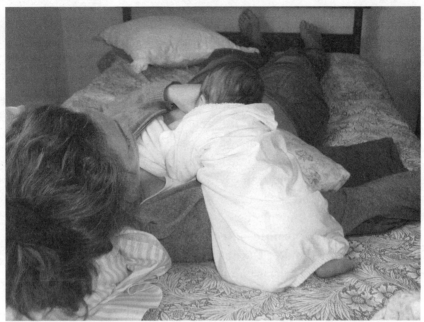

This mother used her creativity to come up with this back-lying breast-feeding position. (©2010 Mary Jane Chase, RNC, MN, CCE, IBCLC, used with permission)

Of course, all new parents know that babies will wake in the night to feed. The great news for you is that, unlike the parents who bottle-feed, you don't have to get out of bed to do it. The trick to this is learning to breastfeed lying down. This allows you to sleep and breastfeed at the same time—what a concept! Once you've mastered that, no one will have to sacrifice rest to feed the baby.

A survival skill. Even if it takes you some practice to master this, don't give up! Breastfeeding lying down can be one of your best coping strategies for the early months. Once you master it, the issue of when your baby will sleep through the night loses much of its significance. Breastfeeding lying down gets easier the more you do it and the older and more coordinated your baby gets.

Practice when awake. When you are first learning, practice during your normal waking hours. We don't know any adults who learn best when they're half asleep. Once you get settled, you can always take a nap. (You probably need one anyway!) But start at a time when you feel awake and alert.

How tos. The most important thing to keep in mind is that, like your breastfeeding rhythm, your way of breastfeeding lying down may be unique. How you feel most comfortable will depend on how you're made. Women have breasts of different sizes and shapes, arms of different lengths, and all sorts of body types. So again, be flexible in your approach. Experiment, experiment, experiment!

When we say "breastfeeding lying down," we're including the semi-reclined, laid-back breastfeeding positions described and illustrated in chapters 1 and 3. Many mothers find these very restful and comfortable. But it's always good to have choices, and some moms prefer to breastfeed on their sides. During the early weeks, side-lying feeding positions are a little trickier and you have to work a little harder at getting a deep latch because gravity pulls your baby's body away from yours. But we include the following details if side-lying breastfeeding is your preference. Consider this description a starting point.

- Start with at least two pillows and a rolled-up hand towel or baby blanket.

- Lie on your side, facing your baby, with a pillow under your head.

- Put the other pillow behind your back.

- Lay your baby completely on her side facing you, and align her body with yours so she is nose to nipple.

- Pull her feet in close to you so your bodies form a V, which may be narrow or wide, depending on your breast size.

- Lean back into the pillow against your back until your nipple lifts off the bed, bringing it to the level of your baby's mouth.

- Put the hand from your upper arm behind your baby's shoulders and pull her gently toward the breast, brushing her mouth and chin lightly against the breast until she opens wide.

- Quickly move her onto the breast by pushing from behind her shoulders to help her get a good, deep latch.

- Press her shoulders tightly against your body as she latches on.

- Wedge the rolled-up towel or baby blanket behind her back to keep her in place, leaving her head free to angle back.

There are many different approaches to breastfeeding on your side, as you will see from the photos in this chapter. Try several until you find one you like. The strategy described above assumes the baby is lying on the bed, but some mothers prefer to rest the baby's head and body on an arm and use that arm to bring the baby onto the breast (see the top photo on page 124). If your baby spits up regularly, you may want to strategically position a bath towel under the two of you that you can easily roll up and replace as needed to avoid having to change sheets.

There are also other ways. For example, mothers of twins often breastfeed at night resting on pillows propped up behind them, tucking a baby under each arm.

When it's time to switch breasts, you also have choices. You can pull your baby against your body, hold her against your upturned chest while you roll over, and begin all over again on the other side. Or you can keep her where she is and lean over to feed from your upper breast (see bottom photo on page 124). One thing's for sure, breastfeeding lying down is worth practicing until you can do it "in your sleep."

SAFE SLEEP

There are few parents who don't sleep with their babies and toddlers at least some of the time, even though our culture and many U.S. health organizations frown on it. Critics of bedsharing are concerned that babies may die if sleeping somewhere besides a crib. One U.S. city actually sent mothers home from the hospital with "never bedshare" magnets—in the shape of coffins! The unfortunate effect of the "never bedshare" edicts by public health organizations is that they inadvertently encourage far more dangerous behaviors in well-meaning parents, such as breastfeeding in the middle of the night on a sofa or recliner, as many mothers have shared with us. Bedsharing can be safe, as studies in countries like Japan have shown. (Japan has one of the lowest SIDS rates in the world, and bedsharing is common.) On the other hand, sleeping with a baby on a sofa or recliner is far more dangerous than sharing a bed. In one recent study of SIDS, sleeping with a baby like this increased the risk of infant death by 66 times (Tappin et al. 2005)!

Yet despite all the dire warnings, a high percentage of families sleep with their babies for at least part of the night. In some households, bedsharing is reserved for special occasions, illness, or naps. In others, parents and babies sleep together on a regular basis. The idea of mothers and babies sleeping separately is actually a relatively recent one, which again coincided with the rise of "scientific mothering" (which we describe in chapter 8).

Mothers don't have to bedshare with their babies in order to breastfeed, but it does make it easier, meaning mothers lose less sleep and get more rest when they do (Quillin and Glenn 2004). In its 2005 policy statement on breastfeeding, the American Academy of Pediatrics recommends that: "Mothers and babies should sleep in proximity to each other to facilitate breastfeeding" (AAP 2005b, 500). And they recommend that babies be in their parents' room for the first six months of life to prevent SIDS. **Note: Just as there are safety standards for cribs and bedding when infants sleep alone, there are also precautions that help ensure safety when mothers and babies sleep together.**

For more on this, see our website (www.breastfeedingmadesimple .com) for the "Guidelines on Co-Sleeping and Breastfeeding" by the Academy of Breastfeeding Medicine (2008). To summarize, this organization of physicians lists the following safe-sleep recommendations:

- Always position babies on their back or side for sleeping.

- Use a firm, flat surface (avoid waterbeds, daybeds, pillows, and loose bedding).

- Don't fall asleep with your baby on a couch, rocker, or recliner. Your baby could fall out of your arms and become trapped or wedged.

- Limit covers for the baby to a thin blanket (no comforters, quilts, duvets, pillows, or stuffed animals near the baby).

- If the room is cold, dress the baby in a warm sleeper.

- Don't leave a baby alone in an adult bed.

- Be sure there are no spaces between the mattress and headboard or walls where a baby could fall or become trapped.

- Also, adults should not share a bed with an infant if they

  - smoke;

  - have consumed alcoholic drinks;

  - are on sedatives or any other drug that impairs awareness.

The Academy of Breastfeeding Medicine also suggests some alternative safe co-sleeping arrangements, such as a firm mattress on the floor away from walls or an infant bed that attaches to the side of an adult bed (or co-sleeper). Many families have found safe and creative ways to meet their own need for sleep while also meeting their baby's need to breastfeed. While keeping these safety recommendations in mind, you are only limited by your imagination!

When the System Breaks Down

Cultural forces have a strong influence on how mothers breastfeed and have much to do with the following practices.

Scheduled Feedings

As mentioned earlier, babies increase a mother's milk production as needed by breastfeeding more often and for longer times. If this can't happen due to scheduled feedings, it puts a mother's milk production and her baby's growth at risk. If a mother's milk production is low at one month, it usually takes much more work for her to raise it. With patience, feeding intervals normally become more predictable and lengthen as babies grow and their stomachs can hold more milk (see chapter 6). For the moment, keep in mind that any attempt to put a baby on a schedule is best left until after the first forty days, when a mother's milk production is set.

Regular Supplements

See chapter 6 for more details on how milk production works, but know for now that whenever your baby receives a supplement, it sends your body the message to make less milk. You cannot increase your milk production by drinking more or eating certain foods. Making milk is all about how many times per day your breasts are well drained. When milk is removed, your body responds by producing more milk. If the milk is not removed (because your baby is full from formula or because you are imposing a feeding schedule), your body slows down milk production. The more times per day and the better drained your breasts are, the more milk you produce. That's how women fully breastfeed twins and triplets (and they do!). They just keep putting baby after baby to the breast, and the breast just keeps making more and more milk.

Some mothers breastfeed with a desire to give their baby both breast and bottle. Even if that is your ultimate goal, consider exclusive breastfeeding for these first forty days. Exclusive breastfeeding puts you in the driver's seat. If you discover your baby has a bad reaction to formula (which is true of 7–8 percent of babies), you have the option of going back to full breastfeeding until your baby outgrows her reaction to nonhuman milks. The mother who hasn't established ample milk production at one month and then discovers that her baby is allergic to formula is in a very different and potentially difficult situation.

Also, regular bottle use can complicate breastfeeding in the beginning. Even if there is expressed mother's milk in the bottle, during these first forty days while a baby is learning to breastfeed, some babies have a difficult time going back and forth between breast and bottle.

This is not true of all babies, and sometimes it can take several bottles before problems develop. Possible problems include breast refusal, ineffective breastfeeding, and suckling changes that cause sore nipples (Righard 1998). Unfortunately, babies aren't born with labels, so you won't know if your baby is susceptible to these kinds of problems until after they occur.

Difficulties are far less likely to happen after the first forty days, once a baby has gotten really practiced at breastfeeding. Despite what you may hear, there is no evidence that waiting until later to give a bottle will make a baby less likely to accept it (Kearney and Cronenwett 1991).

Regular Pacifier Use

Many new parents wonder about using pacifiers. In the same vein, mothers are also frequently cautioned not to let their baby use their breast as a pacifier. We find this odd and even funny! When we are asked about this, our first thought is, "Which came first, the breast or the pacifier?" Of course the pacifier is a breast substitute, not the other way around.

This begs the question: can a baby go to the breast to satisfy her urge to suckle without taking milk? There is no question that a baby can drift off to sleep and suckle very softly at the breast so that no milk is flowing. Of course, there is nothing wrong with this. It's comforting and relaxing to a baby. That's why the pacifier was invented—to provide a baby with exactly this experience without the mother being attached.

The pacifier, however, is not a good tool to use during the first forty days. The purpose of the pacifier is to postpone feedings. It masks baby's feeding cues and throws off a baby's unique feeding rhythm. If it is used often enough, a pacifier can reduce the number of feedings per day during the time baby is working to set your milk production. Once your milk production is well established, a pacifier is less likely to throw a monkey wrench into breastfeeding. During these first forty days, however, it's best to put away the pacifier.

Summary

Every mother and baby pair is different. Breastfeed frequently in these early weeks to set your milk production, and allow your baby to help you do this. Beware of any advice that is the same for all mothers and tries to impose a feeding schedule for you and your baby. Many factors, including your own individual milk storage capacity (the topic of chapter 6), can influence how often your baby needs to feed. Just be sensitive to your baby's cues, and let nature take care of the rest.

CHAPTER 6

Meeting Your Long-Term Breastfeeding Goals

> **Law 6:** *More Milk Out Equals More Milk Made*

How your body makes milk is one of those basic facts of life that every woman should understand, yet few do and misconceptions abound. As we mentioned in chapter 5, the number-one reason women give for weaning their babies earlier than intended is that they are worried about milk production. However, researchers compared a group of mothers who were worried that their babies weren't getting enough milk with a group of unworried mothers and found that both groups of babies were doing well (Hillervik-Lindquist, Hofvander, and Sjölin 1991).

This is definitely a case where knowledge is power. Your understanding of milk production makes it possible for you to make feeding choices consistent with your long-term breastfeeding goals. Part of this includes understanding how individual differences affect milk production and feeding patterns. Another part is knowing where you fall within the spectrum of normal so that you can take this into account as you make your choices. This is especially important if you and your baby are not average, or near the center of this spectrum. One of our goals in this chapter is to share with you some of the new information that strips away the mystery so that you will know how to adjust your milk production as needed.

The Reward Period

But let's begin by describing this new phase in your life with your baby. As you leave the newborn period, breastfeeding becomes much easier—easier, in fact, than bottlefeeding. But there are other issues requiring your attention. With a new baby in your family, your life has changed forever. And as you leave the "mommy zone" of the first forty days and emerge with your baby into the outside world, you and your household must adjust to the new routines that are inevitable when a new member joins your family.

Breastfeeding Is Easier

At around six weeks or so, you and your baby move out of the newborn adjustment period and into the reward period. Feedings are easier, because with practice and growth, breastfeeding becomes easy and automatic. Your baby has more head and neck control, so attachment is easier in all feeding positions. Your baby is a much more active participant. Mothers who had worried about breastfeeding away from home because they needed a special chair or a special pillow now find that they are breastfeeding while walking around the house and that they can easily breastfeed no matter where they are. Breastfeeding lying down becomes a simple matter. A helper and dim lighting are no longer needed for night feedings, because if your baby is laid anywhere near the breast, he latches himself on quickly.

This is the time, as we explained in chapter 5, when breastfeeding becomes easier than the alternative. No one needs to be awake and alert to handle night feedings. There is no mixing, no shopping, no bottle washing, no clogged nipples during feedings, and no worries about running out of formula. (As of this writing, finding formula is a real concern for bottlefeeding mothers in Haiti, who are dealing with the aftermath of a catastrophic earthquake.)

Your Breastfeeding Goals

If you have followed your baby's feeding rhythm and allowed him to set your milk production during those first forty days, you will most likely have full milk production as you move into the reward period, which simply means that your baby is gaining weight normally without the use of formula. This puts you in an enviable position. You can decide where you want to go from here. And your possibilities are nearly unlimited. Let's review some of your choices.

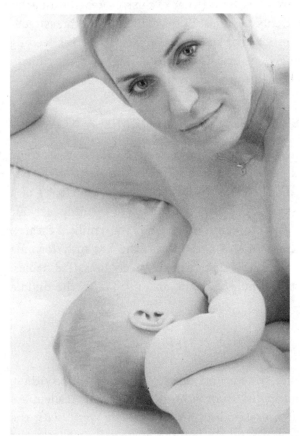

In the reward period, breastfeeding gets much easier.

IF YOU WEAN NOW

You've given your baby six weeks of normal gut function and normal immune-system growth during the most vulnerable time of his life. Keep in mind that, from your baby's perspective, the longer you can delay introducing any formula, the better. Cow's milk (the basis for most infant formulas) is the most common *allergen*, or allergy trigger, out there for humans. IgA antibodies (one of the many living components of your breast milk) prevent the absorption of allergens like cow's milk proteins through your baby's gut and into his bloodstream. By restricting these allergens to the gut, they are less likely to pass intact into the bloodstream and trigger an allergic reaction. It takes about six months for a baby's gut to start producing IgA antibodies on its own, which is one reason delaying solid foods until six months is recommended and why research has found that exclusive breastfeeding for the first six months prevents allergies. But even if you stop breastfeeding now, there is no question that six weeks of exclusive breastfeeding is better than none and gives your baby's digestive system some time to mature before being exposed to the allergens of nonhuman milks.

IF YOU CHOOSE TO GIVE SOME FORMULA NOW

When making feeding choices, also keep in mind that some human milk is always better than none. If you choose to give your baby both your milk and formula, the health risks to your baby of a partial weaning are less than the risks of a complete weaning, as your baby will continue to get some antibodies from your milk. Research has found that at four months of age, babies who are fully formula fed have twice as many ear infections as exclusively breastfed babies. The babies getting both formula and human milk fall in the middle (Duncan et al. 1993).

IF YOU EXCLUSIVELY BREASTFEED

Your baby's immune system and digestive system will continue to grow and develop normally. The reason the American Academy of Pediatrics recommends breastfeeding for at least one year (with the addition of solid foods at around six months) is because research has found that for normal immune-system function later in life, we need to receive those living components of human milk for a minimum of twelve months (AAP 2005b).

However, whether your ultimate breastfeeding goal is six weeks, three months, six months, twelve months, or beyond, to meet your goal, you need to understand the physical laws in place and how to use these laws in your favor. And you need to figure out how to make breastfeeding work within the context of your daily life. (See chapter 9 for tips for making this easier.)

How Milk Production Works

As we mentioned in the beginning of this chapter, there are basic facts of life concerning milk production that every woman should know. Understanding these dynamics gives you both more control over your breastfeeding experience and more satisfaction. When you know how milk production works, you will spend less time worrying and more time relaxing and enjoying your baby.

There are two main dynamics at work in Law 6 (*More milk out equals more milk made*): *degree of breast fullness,* or how full your breasts are, and *breast storage capacity,* or how much milk your breasts hold at their fullest time during the day.

Degree of Breast Fullness

Our knowledge about milk production increased dramatically during the 1990s and early 2000s due to the work of a Western Australian research team led by Dr. Peter Hartmann. The Hartmann team, with the help of local breastfeeding volunteers, used a high-tech approach to learn more about how the breast makes milk. In some of their studies they used techniques from the field of topography, which measures mountain terrains, to chart physical changes in the breast and determine how much milk the breasts hold (Cregan and Hartmann 1999). They used ultrasensitive scales to weigh babies before and after feedings to determine exactly how much milk a baby takes at each breast, at each feeding, and over a twenty-four-hour period (Daly,

Owens, and Hartmann 1993). And they used ultrasound to observe internal breast changes during feedings (Ramsay et al. 2004).

Their findings have taught us that one of the primary factors that affects how quickly or slowly milk is made is the degree of breast fullness (how full the breasts are).

THE FACTORY ANALOGY

To understand more clearly how this concept works, imagine a factory that makes widgets:

- *Low demand equals slow production.* As you enter the factory, you're told that widget sales are slow. You notice stacks of widgets everywhere. Orders for widgets are few and far between, and as you watch, the stacks of widgets grow. With production greater than demand, it's obvious that the workers on the widget assembly line feel no sense of urgency. As the stacks of widgets grow higher, the workers work more and more slowly.

- *High demand equals faster production.* Now imagine that a radical upswing in business occurs. Suddenly widget sales are on the rise. The stacks of widgets in the factory begin to shrink and then vanish. Fewer widgets are available to fill orders, which continue to come in at a faster and faster clip. As demand exceeds production, the workers work faster and faster to keep up with widget sales.

Full breasts make milk slower. The same thing happens within the breast. As the breast becomes full, production slows down. Why does this happen? Scientists tell us this slow-down is due to a combination of the pressure the milk exerts within the breast and a substance in the milk called *feedback inhibitor of lactation*, or FIL for short (Prentice 1989). FIL sends a signal to your breasts to decrease the rate of milk production. As the amount of milk in your breasts increases, so does the amount of FIL. The more FIL in your breasts, the stronger the signal to slow milk production. As your breasts get fuller and fuller, like the factory filling with widgets, your rate of milk production slows down.

Drained breasts make milk faster. The opposite is also true. The Hartmann team found that milk production speeds up when a mother's breasts are drained more fully (Daly et al. 1996). If a baby needs to adjust his mother's milk production, this is how he does it: he feeds more often and he breastfeeds longer, taking a larger percentage of the available milk. As we explained in previous chapters, the milk a baby gets as he drains the breast also has increased fat content. So even if there is just a little milk left in the breast, as he continues to breastfeed, he will get more of the "high-octane" fatty milk. A little of this fatty milk goes a long way toward leaving baby satisfied. (Think "chocolate éclair"!)

Ever hear someone say, "You need to let your breasts fill up before you feed the baby"? Anyone who says this is seriously confused about how milk production works.

What's average? To better understand the concept of degree of breast fullness, it helps to know what's average. Although many mothers assume that babies take all of their available milk when they breastfeed, the Hartmann team found otherwise. Their research indicates that on average, babies take about 67 percent of the milk in the breasts (Kent 2007). This means that at an average feeding, 33 percent (or one third) of the milk is left in the breasts. If a mother wants to increase her rate of milk production, in addition to increasing the number of feedings, she can drain her breasts more fully. This can be done in one of two ways:

- Have baby breastfeed on each breast more than once during each feeding, if he is willing.

- Express milk after the feeding.

The bottom line is: The more drained a mother's breasts are at the end of a feeding and the more times a day they are well drained, the faster her breasts will make milk.

Lopsided? The Hartmann team's research also tells us clearly that milk production, while influenced by hormones in the beginning, is most greatly influenced over the long term by milk removal (breastfeeding or pumping) and confirms that each breast regulates its own production (Kent 2007). In our experience, it is not at all unusual for milk production to vary between breasts, sometimes considerably. Research has found this to be more common than not (Hill et al. 2007). This can happen if, like many mothers, you find breastfeeding on one side more comfortable and tend to favor that side. And it can happen if one of your breasts is just naturally a larger milk producer.

You may not realize there is a difference in production unless you pump or unless the difference is so marked that you look lopsided. But ultimately, it doesn't matter. This is not a permanent change. When your baby weans, your breasts will return to being the same size again. What's most important is that your baby gets enough milk overall, not whether he gets exactly the same amount of milk from each breast.

Breast Storage Capacity

The concept of degree of breast fullness sounds simple enough, but there is also one other recently discovered factor at work that is a major player in your milk production. Have you ever heard that breast size has no bearing on your ability to breastfeed? Well that is true, but the Hartmann team found that the storage space within the milk-making (or glandular) tissue in your breast can affect your baby's feeding patterns (Kent et al. 2006). This second factor, breast storage capacity, goes a long way toward explaining why feeding rhythms vary so much from one mother-baby pair to another.

Breast storage capacity simply refers to the most milk your breasts hold during the day. This is not related to breast size, as size is usually determined more by the amount of fatty tissue in the breasts. This means that smaller-breasted mothers with more room in their glandular tissue can still have a large storage capacity and hold large amounts of milk.

LARGE STORAGE CAPACITY

A mother with a large storage capacity will likely notice a far different breastfeeding rhythm during months one through six as compared with the mother with a small storage capacity. A mother's breast storage capacity affects feeding patterns in several ways.

One breast or two? A mother's storage capacity can affect whether her baby usually takes one breast or two at each feeding. Why is that? Think back to the degree-of-breast-fullness dynamic. A full breast makes milk slower, and a drained breast makes milk faster. Let's say a mother with a large storage capacity holds 5 oz. (150 ml) of milk in each breast. Let's also say that a three-month-old baby whose stomach has grown and stretched can now comfortably hold 5 oz. (150 ml) of milk. First, as mentioned in chapter 4, babies usually take one breast at some feedings and both breasts at other feedings. Many mothers with a large storage capacity report that their babies almost always take one breast at a feeding and have no interest in taking the other breast when it's offered. This is because the baby always gets enough milk from one breast to satisfy him.

If a baby always takes only one breast at each feeding, that means there may be long stretches of time before each breast is drained. For example, if the baby takes the right breast at 2 p.m. and the left breast at 5 p.m., there may be six hours or more between drainings. But because a mother with a large storage capacity can hold more milk, her milk production will not drop as a result. In fact, spacing out feedings this way will probably prevent the opposite problem—an overly abundant milk production. If a mother makes far more milk than her baby needs, the baby may have difficulty handling the fast milk flow. Too much milk can also be a challenge to the mother, because she may be more prone to problems such as *mastitis* (infection of the breast).

Number of feedings per day. A large storage capacity can also have a major effect on the number of feedings per day. Many mothers are surprised to learn that due to baby's slowing growth rate, his total daily milk intake remains remarkably stable from one to six months of age. At around one month, a breastfed baby reaches his peak daily milk intake of about 25–35 oz. (750–1,050 ml) of milk per day, and this stays roughly the same until he begins solid foods at six months and his need for milk decreases as his solids intake increases.

At one month, the average baby's stomach comfortably holds about 4 oz. (120 ml) of milk, so to get enough milk during the course of the day, he needs to breastfeed, on average, about eight times. (Multiply feedings by ounces—8 × 4—to get 32 oz. [960 ml] per day.) But as he grows and his stomach grows and stretches, the amount of milk he can take at each breastfeeding increases.

A mother with a large storage capacity has more than 4 oz. (120 ml) available at each feeding, and as her baby grows, he may begin to take more milk, say 5–6 oz. (150–180 ml), at a feeding. If this happens, it will, of course, change his feeding pattern. Since the amount of milk he needs in a day stays the same, if he increases his milk intake at feedings, his number of feedings per day will go down. In other words, the baby who previously needed to breastfeed eight times per day to get 25–35 oz. (750–1,050 ml) per day now needs to feed only six times per day to get about the same amount of milk. (As above, multiply feedings by ounces—6 × 5.3—to get the same 32 oz. [960 ml] per day.)

Obviously, the mother we mentioned in chapter 5, whose chunky baby fed five times per day, had a very large storage capacity.

Of course, as we described in that same chapter, milk production ebbs and flows over the course of the day, so a baby will not always take the same amount of milk at every feeding. But hopefully this example clarifies this idea.

Effect on sleeping patterns. Taking more milk per feeding may also affect a baby's need to wake at night to feed. The baby who needs fewer feedings per day tends to sleep through the night at an earlier age than other babies. Yet even with longer stretches between feedings at night, a mother with a large storage capacity may not become uncomfortably full by morning since her breasts hold more milk. This means she can maintain her milk production in spite of these longer stretches.

SMALL STORAGE CAPACITY

Now let's look at the other side of the coin. The most important point to remember is that women with a small storage capacity produce plenty of milk for their babies. Researchers noted that none of the women in their studies with a small storage capacity had a problem with low milk production or slow weight gain in their babies (Kent et al. 2006); their babies were thriving. But these mother-baby pairs had a different feeding rhythm. Let's see what changes.

One breast or two? If the baby of a mother with an average storage capacity takes one breast at some feedings and both breasts at some feedings, what is typical for a mother with a small storage capacity? In general, these babies want both breasts at almost every feeding, especially by one month of age or so, when they can take more milk.

Let's say a mother with a small storage capacity can hold 2 oz. (60 ml) in each breast. At one month, her baby needs to breastfeed eight or nine times per day to get the 25–35 oz. (750–1,050 ml) per day he needs. (Multiply two breasts by ounces by feedings—2 × 2 × 8—to get 32 oz. [945 ml] per day.) What is different, however, is that during months one through six, his milk intake per feeding will not change. Unlike the pair in which the mother has a large storage capacity, this mother's breasts hold 2 oz. (60 ml) apiece. So, no matter how big the baby's stomach gets, he will get no more than 4 oz. (120 ml) per feeding.

Number of feedings per day. This individual difference has a profound effect on a baby's daily feeding pattern. To find out how, let's do the math. A baby continues to need 25–35 oz. (750–1,050 ml) per day. He can take a maximum of 4 oz. (120 ml) of milk per feeding. What will happen if his mother attempts to drop some feedings as he grows? (This is sometimes recommended on the premise that older babies don't "need" as many breastfeedings.) Dropping feedings affects this baby in two ways:

1. The baby's overall milk intake per day goes down, because it is impossible for the baby to take more milk at each feeding to make up for the dropped feeding(s).

2. The mother's milk production slows.

With fewer feedings, the baby's weight gain will likely slow or stop. Depending on the number of feedings dropped, he may even lose weight. A baby in this situation will be underfed, which means he'll probably also be understandably fussy and unhappy. His sleep may suffer, as well.

The mother with a small storage capacity is also at risk for slowed milk production. Why? When a mother drops a feeding, this means the intervals between feedings increase. Remember, full breasts make milk slower and drained breasts make milk faster. A mother whose breasts can hold 2 oz. (60 ml) will feel full very quickly in comparison with the mother whose breasts can hold 5 oz. (150 ml). If she decides it's time to train her baby to sleep through the night and subsequently goes seven or eight hours between feedings, her breasts will become hard and full after four or five hours. Not only does that put her at risk for mastitis, but her full breasts will make milk slower. She gives her body the signal to slow down her milk production.

As long as a mother with a small storage capacity continues to feed her baby when the baby shows hunger cues, and continues feeding enough times per day, her milk production will be fine. (The exact number of feedings needed will vary according to storage capacity.) But if she stretches out the time between feedings or drops them to the point that her breasts feel full, her body will respond by producing less milk. She will know she has reached a critical threshold when her baby's weight gain falters.

Effect on sleeping patterns. It is the mother with a small storage capacity whose baby continues to wake and breastfeed every few hours during the night. Continued night feedings are normal for this mother and baby. The baby needs them to get enough milk, and the mother needs them to keep up her milk production. If this mother has a breastfeeding goal of twelve months, she needs to plan to continue night feedings. (As we explained in chapter 4, many families get creative with strategies for getting their sleep while continuing to breastfeed at night.)

What Is Full Milk Production?

Now that you understand some of the most basic dynamics of milk production, let's discuss a foolproof way to know if you have enough milk: you simply check your baby's weight gain.

Normal Weight Gain

No matter what else is happening with breastfeeding (feeding patterns, sleep patterns, fussy times, etc.), if you are exclusively breastfeeding and your baby is gaining weight normally, you have full milk production.

It also helps to know that normal weight gain has different definitions at different ages. Babies' weight gain slows down as they get older, because their growth also slows down. If a baby continued to gain and grow at his newborn pace throughout his life, he would grow into a giant.

Another point to understand is that until recently our standard growth charts were based on the weight gains of babies on formula, which research found to be slightly different from breastfeeding norms (WHO 2006). The numbers below are based on populations of breastfed babies, and they reflect average weight gains (not minimally acceptable weight gains). These numbers provide a reliable guide to how breastfeeding is going.

Birth to four days	Loss of up to 7–10 percent of birth weight
Four days to four months	Gain of 7–8 oz. (200–225 g) per week (2 lbs./0.91 kg per month)
Four to six months	Gain of 4–5 oz./113–142 g per week (1 lb./0.45 kg per month)
Six to twelve months	Gain of 3–4 oz./85–113 g per week (12 oz./0.34 kg per month)

If you're exclusively breastfeeding, you may want to ask your baby's health care provider if the growth chart he or she uses is the chart from the World Health Organization based on breastfeeding norms.

If not, it will not accurately measure healthy growth. If your baby's weight gain is less than the table above, see chapter 10 for strategies for increasing it.

WEIGHT CHECKS

What should you do if you are worried about whether your baby is getting enough milk? (In our culture, it can be hard not to be worried with all the second-guessing that well-meaning people around us do.) That's simple. Call your baby's health care provider and make an appointment to have your baby weighed.

Knowing your baby's weight gain will address your concern. If it turns out that your baby is doing well, you can relax and stop worrying. If you find out your baby's weight is of concern, you can seek skilled breastfeeding help right away. If there is a problem, the sooner you make adjustments, the easier it is to get breastfeeding back on track.

YOUR BABY'S DIAPERS

In chapters 4 and 5, we talked about how you can use your baby's stools as an indicator of how breastfeeding is going. As your baby gets older, this is not as reliable. After about six weeks, some babies cut down on their output of stools yet still gain and grow well. If this happens with your baby, it makes sense to get his weight checked to confirm this is normal for him. But it is definitely not a cause for panic.

Common Misconceptions

If your baby is exclusively breastfeeding and has a weight in the normal range, there is no doubt that your milk production is more than adequate. Remember, at each feeding baby only takes, on average, about 67 percent of the milk in the breasts. That means there is plenty of milk over and above what your baby is taking. Even so, many mothers worry. What are their worries? These worries about milk production most often reflect general confusion about normal breastfeeding. Mothers' concerns fall into two main categories: worries about the baby and worries about their breasts.

BABY FALSE ALARMS

Because most new mothers today have not had much exposure to normal breastfeeding, they may mistakenly interpret any of the following baby behaviors as signs that they don't have enough milk:

- Baby seems hungry sooner than expected (adjust expectations).

- Baby wants to feed more often and/or longer (normal during a growth spurt).

- Baby suddenly breastfeeds for a shorter time (babies get faster with practice).

- Baby is fussy (almost all babies—no matter how they're fed—have fussy periods).

As we've discussed in the chapters 4 and 5, these can all be part of normal breastfeeding.

Some mothers attempt to "test" breastfeeding by giving the baby a bottle after breastfeeding. Their thinking is that if the baby takes milk from the bottle, it proves that their milk production is low. However, bottle nipples tend to flow fast and—unlike the breast—consistently, so many babies will take milk from the bottle even if they have had enough from the breast. It is always possible to overfeed a baby with a bottle because of its fast and consistent flow. Formula, and even your milk in a bottle, stimulate your baby to eat. However, he's not eating because he is hungry, but simply because the bottle's fast flow triggers his sucking reflex.

Another test involves weighing the baby before and after a breastfeeding. Unfortunately, most scales (including those available from baby stores) are not accurate enough to detect the small differences between the before and after weights. As we mentioned before, it is even less accurate to weigh yourself on the bathroom scale, weigh yourself again while holding your baby, and then subtract the difference. Scales are available, however, that are accurate enough to measure babies intake at the breast (see our Resources section for information on how to find these). But don't make assumptions about your baby's milk intake at the breast without using the right equipment.

MOTHER FALSE ALARMS

Mothers also worry when they notice the following changes in themselves, but bear in mind that these are also false alarms:

- Breasts seem softer (this is normal at about two to three weeks).

- Breasts aren't leaking (some mothers never leak; others stop eventually).

- Don't feel a milk release or let-down (it can happen without your knowing).

- Can't express much milk (this is a learned skill, not a test of milk production).

COUNTERPRODUCTIVE STRATEGIES

Then there are the strategies recommended to women that are simply wrong-headed and cause unnecessary worry and breastfeeding problems.

Misconception	Fact
Wait until your breasts refill before feeding again.	Full breasts make milk slower.
Follow a one-size-fits-all feeding schedule.	Differences in breast storage capacities mean one feeding rhythm will not work well for all mothers and babies.
Measure your milk production by pumping instead of breastfeeding.	Milk expression is a learned skill, and the Hartmann team found that 10 percent of the women whose babies were doing very well at the breast were unable to pump milk effectively (Mitoulas et al. 2002).

What Everyone Thinks Affects Milk Production (But Doesn't)

Misconceptions about milk production abound, even among health professionals. When women ask what they can do to increase their milk production, the following are usually the first suggestions given:

- Drink more fluids.

- Eat a better diet.

- Get more rest.

Yet except under extreme conditions, these have little to no effect on milk production.

Drink More Fluids

When you ask what to do to increase milk production, chances are this will be the first response you get, and it seems logical. After all, a breastfeeding mother's body loses slightly less than a liter of fluid a day via her milk. However, research has found no connection between fluid intake and milk production. In fact, one study found that when mothers force fluids (drink more than they feel inclined to), they had a slight decrease in milk production (Dusdieker et al. 1985). (You read that right!) What is recommended for the breastfeeding mother is simply to "drink to thirst." There is no advantage to drinking more.

Eat a Better Diet

Of course, it's always good to eat a healthy diet. When a mother eats well, she feels better. She has more energy and more resistance to illness. These are good things and should be encouraged. But they aren't the same as increasing her milk production. A mother's body is made to provide first for her baby. When mothers in developing countries were studied, researchers found that it took famine conditions for three weeks or longer before the quality or quantity of their milk was affected (Prentice et al. 1983). In developed countries, unless a mother is in extreme poverty or has an eating disorder, improving her diet will probably have little or no effect on milk production.

Get More Rest

Just like a nutritious diet, adequate rest is always a plus in terms of a mother's energy and resistance to illness, but no connection has been found between rest (or lack thereof) and milk production. Besides, if need be, a tired mother can sleep while she breastfeeds.

You may think that drinking more fluids, improving diet, and getting more rest are harmless enough, even if they don't have the desired effect, but unfortunately, many women assume that if they have tried them, they have done "everything possible." Then, when these efforts don't improve their production, they end up feeling that their only alternative is to give formula. Another drawback is that mothers may spend a considerable amount of time and effort on improving nutrition and resting that would be better spent improving their breastfeeding dynamics and increasing the number of feedings. Focusing on these other things leaves women essentially spinning their wheels in their effort to increase their milk production.

Meeting Your Long-Term Goals

You now have much of the information you need to meet your long-term breastfeeding goals. But there are still a few more points that may help you.

How to Think About Breastfeeding

As you gain confidence in your milk production and your baby's feeding effectiveness, you will probably become more aware of the emotional aspects of breastfeeding. Once you know that the nutrition part of breastfeeding is covered, you can focus on the closeness and comfort it gives you and your baby. We discussed the amazing impact of skin-to-skin contact in chapter 2 and the relaxing and relationship-building effects of the hormone oxytocin, which is released every time you breastfeed. Research also indicates that breastfeeding mothers are less stressed than bottlefeeding mothers, no doubt in part due to the hormones of breastfeeding and the extra skin-to-skin contact (Heinrichs, Neumann, and Ehlert 2002).

While breastfeeding is a vital source of nutrition for your baby, it is also much more than a feeding method. It's a wonderful way to calm and comfort your baby, to make the transition to sleep easier, and to cement that vital first relationship between mother and baby that sets the tone for your baby's emotional life. In so many ways, breastfeeding is a remarkably effective mothering tool.

NUMBER OF FEEDINGS PER DAY

Some parents worry that allowing a baby to feed whenever he shows an interest might cause overfeeding. One thing we know for sure: a mother cannot "make" a baby breastfeed, which makes worries about overfeeding unnecessary. In fact, as we mentioned in chapter 4, studies indicate that breastfed babies are 25 percent less likely to be obese than their bottlefed counterparts (Armstrong and Reilly 2002). The properties of human milk no doubt play a part, as well as the baby's ability to self-regulate feedings at the breast, which teaches healthy eating habits. Unlike bottlefeeding, a breastfeeding mother cannot see what is left in the breast, so there is no temptation to "tank baby up" to keep him full longer or to avoid waste.

In addition, it is impossible for a mother to breastfeed to meet her own "selfish" needs, an accusation leveled by the uneducated and inexperienced. Yet it is also true that with breastfeeding, there is always more going on than just feeding. Whether a baby wants to breastfeed for thirst (taking only the thin, watery foremilk), hunger (breastfeeding long enough to get to the fattier milk), comfort (to ease feelings of fear or loneliness), or closeness (because he loves you!) is immaterial. Any and all of these needs are legitimately met at the breast and have been for as long as humans have breastfed. You don't need to worry about your baby's reasons when you put him to breast. Breastfeeding is the ultimate in multitasking! As one mother of an older baby said, "I don't count breastfeedings any more than I count kisses." Breastfeeding is a way to give and receive love as well as a way to feed, which is one reason this is called the reward period. This is when the loving aspect of breastfeeding comes to the forefront.

AMOUNT OF MILK BABIES NEED

As we've explained, research tells us that breastfed babies from one to six months take an average of 25–35 oz. (750–1,050 ml) a day (Neville et al. 1988). When this amount was first discovered, it caused concern, because that is significantly less than the amount of formula bottlefed babies consume.

Human milk vs. formula intake. Research has found that at the age of four months, babies on formula take on average about 33 percent more milk per day than breastfed babies (Neville et al. 1988). This fact has been confirmed many times over, so we know that it's true. This difference in intake is good to know, because sometimes breastfeeding mothers assume they need to pump as much milk for a feeding as their formula-feeding friends' babies take from the bottle—not so.

Why is this? Some research indicates that the breastfed baby digests his food more efficiently than the baby on formula. One U.S. study concluded that "formula-fed infants are almost twofold less efficient than breastfed infants in their utilization of dietary nitrogen..." (Motil et al. 1997, 15). This means that formula-fed babies need more calories just to maintain normal function. Because formula is made from nonhuman milks, a baby's system cannot use it as completely, so he needs more of it for adequate nutrition.

Effect of the delivery system. Another factor that affects how much milk a baby drinks is the milk delivery system, in other words, whether baby is fed by breast or bottle. We have observed that babies fed human milk by bottle tend to feed with the same pattern as babies who take formula by bottle. They take more at a feeding and feed fewer times per day. In the beginning, breastfed babies tend to average eight to twelve feedings per day, while bottlefed babies (no matter what's in the bottle) average more like six to eight feedings per day.

Why is this? As adults, we are advised by experts to eat slowly so that our appetite control mechanism takes effect. What this means is that when you eat slowly, you feel full with less food. Conversely, when you eat fast, you tend to overeat because the signals from your stomach have not caught up with the signals to your brain.

The same thing seems to be true for babies. In general, milk comes faster from the bottle, which has a continuous flow. Babies tend to have more control over milk flow from the breast, which flows faster and slower with milk releases. Dietitians tell adults that the healthiest eating pattern is many small meals over the course of a day. Breastfeeding teaches this healthy eating habit from birth. Bottlefeeding, on the other hand, teaches a baby to overfeed (Kramer et al. 2004).

For breastfeeding mothers who use bottles regularly, this is important to know. This means you do not need to panic if your baby takes more from a bottle than the amount of milk you can pump at one sitting. If you know that your baby is likely to take more from the bottle than the breast, then you will know that this is not a sign of a low milk production. If this happens, chalk it up to the difference in the delivery system.

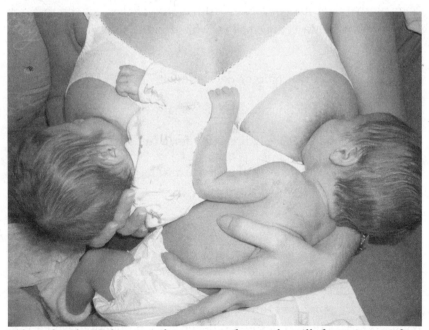

When they know how, mothers can make ample milk for twins, triplets, and even quadruplets. (©2005 Catherine Watson Genna, BS, IBCLCs, used with permission)

151

It may be our cultural familiarity with bottles that is at the root of the erroneous advice given to breastfeeding mothers to drop feedings as their babies get older. Just as mothers of an earlier era were motivated to toilet train their babies within the first year to lighten laundry loads, eliminating feedings by tanking babies up on the bottle helps to eliminate some of the housekeeping work of bottlefeeding. However, with no bottles to wash and no formula to prepare, this is not an issue for a breastfeeding mother.

Starting Solid Foods

We will discuss solid foods in more detail in chapter 7, but know, for now, that the old recommendation of starting solid foods at four to six months has been revised. The World Health Organization convened a panel of experts to examine all the available research on the ideal age for starting solids, and in 2001 they published their conclusion: delaying solids until six months results in better health outcomes for both mothers and babies (WHO 2001). This analysis of the research revealed that breastfeeding babies who delayed solid foods until six months

- had better neuromotor development;

- had less infectious disease, especially diarrhea.

Mothers who exclusively breastfed for a full six months

- had a longer delay in their return to fertility;

- had a faster weight loss.

When you begin giving solid foods can also affect your ability to meet your long-term breastfeeding goals because solid foods take the place of milk in your baby's diet. When solids are given too early, you replace a more age-appropriate food with a food that will fill your baby up but that he cannot yet fully digest. The earlier solids are started, the higher the risks of allergies and reduced milk production, which may undermine your long-term goals.

When the System Breaks Down

The following are common choices mothers sometimes make without realizing they may undermine their long-term breastfeeding goals.

Scheduled or Dropped Feedings

The "Breast Storage Capacity" section (earlier in this chapter) explains why scheduled or dropped feedings decrease milk production and thwart some mothers' efforts to meet their breastfeeding goals. Let's look at what happened to one mother in this situation to see how this happens (all too often) in real life.

Gabrielle called a lactation consultant because she was in a quandary. She had been breastfeeding her son Ben for six months but had been struggling with her milk production since he was two months old. Ben was a sleepy baby from the start and had slept long ten-to-twelve-hour stretches at night. At first he breastfed eight to ten times per day, and Gabrielle knew this was normal for a newborn.

But everywhere Gabrielle turned, she heard or read that she should cut back on feedings as Ben got older. So when she started work at two months, she began to cut back. Almost immediately her milk production dropped. The first thing she did was to get up in the night to pump her milk, because she didn't want to wake her sleeping baby. For a month she gave him this extra milk and was able to continue to exclusively breastfeed. But as she continued to drop feedings, she also dropped the nightly pumping. By four months, Ben was breastfeeding five times per day and needing more milk than she could pump at work, so she began giving him formula as well.

Gabrielle tried some of the milk-increasing tricks she had heard about, for a while taking fenugreek capsules and later getting her doctor to prescribe metoclopramide, a drug that increases milk production in some mothers. Every time she used one of these tricks, her milk production would increase and she would go back to exclusive breastfeeding, but once she stopped, her production slowed again.

The lactation consultant explained degree of breast fullness and milk storage capacity, and Gabrielle realized that she had a small storage capacity. She also understood now what was going wrong. Her strategy of dropping feedings as Ben grew older was working against her. She had a breastfeeding goal of one year, and she still wanted to achieve it. What did she decide to do? She increased her number of breastfeedings at home and pumpings at work and started getting up at night to pump again. (She could have awakened Ben for the night feeding, but she decided she'd rather let him sleep.) Meeting her breastfeeding goal was important to her, and now that she knew how to reach it, she adjusted her routine to make it happen.

Too Much Solid Food Too Soon

In some cases, solid foods started too early and too enthusiastically have drastically reduced mothers' milk production and short-circuited their long-term breastfeeding goals. See chapter 7 for strategies to help your baby transition to solid foods in the best possible way and at the best possible time.

Summary

Once full milk production is established, the number of times per day a mother needs to drain her breasts to maintain milk production can vary greatly, depending on individual differences. New research on breast storage capacity has been able to answer questions about why babies have such different feeding patterns. It also gives us some explanation for why babies differ on when they start sleeping through the night and why imposing feeding schedules can be a very bad idea for some mothers and babies.

CHAPTER 7

Weaning Comfortably and Happily

> **Law 7:** *Children Wean Naturally*

Weaning is one of the few experiences that all breastfeeding mothers share. In the United States, weaning means completely stopping breastfeeding. It begins when your baby takes food or drink other than your milk and ends with the last breastfeeding. In the United Kingdom and other countries throughout the world, weaning means adding other foods besides mother's milk. In this chapter, we are primarily using weaning to mean cessation of breastfeeding. But we will also be discussing the introduction of solids as a form of weaning.

Although you may think of weaning as an event, it is actually a process. Weaning may be your choice or your child's choice, or it may be mutual. It may be abrupt or gradual, taking days, weeks, months, or even years.

A Weaning Overview

The word "wean" is derived from a word meaning "satisfaction" or "fulfillment." During most of history, weaning was considered a natural stage of growth, a sign that a child had finally had her fill and was ready to move away from her mother and into the wider world. King David described the sense of fulfillment and inner peace a child gains when weaning comes in its own time when he wrote in Psalm 131:2: "Surely I have stilled and quieted my soul; Like a weaned child with his mother, Like a weaned child is my soul within me."

In the United States today, however, weaning is not seen as a process to be celebrated or a naturally occurring stage of growth. Weaning is commonly considered a time of deprivation and unhappiness. It is the approach to weaning, however, that makes the difference. A rigid and abrupt approach makes weaning painful and difficult. But this does not have to be. There are ways to wean that are as gentle and loving as the way breastfeeding began. Weaning gradually—with consideration for the feelings and preferences of both mother and child—can make it the positive experience we'd all like it to be. And that's what this chapter is all about.

When to Wean

Every family makes its own decision about when to wean. This is as it should be, because every family is unique and has its own considerations. As you weigh the relevant factors for you and your family, it may help you to know what the experts say about age of weaning and why.

WHAT THE EXPERTS SAY

According to the American Academy of Pediatrics,

Breastfeeding should be continued for at least the first year of life and beyond for as long as mutually desired by mother and child (AAP 2005b).

Why is breastfeeding recommended "for at least the first year of life" by the American Academy of Pediatrics, the group that advises pediatricians on good practice? After reviewing the research, its expert panel found that duration of breastfeeding had a significant impact on the lifelong health of children. Studies indicate that the living properties of human milk are needed for at least one year for there to be a measurable effect on the incidence of immune-related illnesses later in life, such as Crohn's disease, Hodgkin's disease, leukemia, ulcerative colitis, and others (AAP 2005b). The long-term health outcomes of babies weaned younger than one year were measurably worse. The research that they cited in support of this recommendation was a study of a group of American mothers who ignored cultural norms and whose babies weaned, on average, from two-and-a-half to three years of age (Sugarman and Kendall-Tackett 1995).

Another research-based recommendation comes from the World Health Organization (WHO). WHO's role is to provide international public-health guidelines. WHO serves developed nations, such as the United States, as well as developing countries, where in many areas the risks of illness and death are higher due to sanitation problems, fluctuating food and water supplies, and lack of available health care.

> [E]xclusive breastfeeding for 6 months is the optimal way of feeding infants. Thereafter infants should receive complementary foods with continued breastfeeding up to 2 years of age or beyond (WHO 2001).

WHO's recommendation of "two years and beyond" is based on research in developing and developed countries into health outcomes of children older than one year (Goldman, Garza, and Goldblum 1983). These studies found that even when children are weaned after one year of age, they are at greater risk for illness and death. Weaned children between sixteen and thirty-six months of age have more types of illnesses of longer duration and need more medical care than breastfeeding children the same age (Gulick 1986). Weaned children twelve to thirty-six months old were three-and-a-half times more likely to die than those still breastfeeding (Molbak et al. 1994).

There is no doubt that the living antibodies in human milk work their magic as long as your child receives your milk. This is important for a toddler, because even with the help provided by human milk, some aspects of her immune system will not fully function on their own for eighteen months, while other aspects take as long as five to six years to fully develop. This timing is not coincidental, as historical and cross-cultural perspectives on breastfeeding indicate.

A Brief History of Weaning

In the United States, babies tend to be weaned young. Statistics for 2006 from the U.S. Centers for Disease Control and Prevention tell us that by six months, 57 percent of American babies are not breastfeeding. By one year, 77 percent have weaned (CDC 2010).

But before you make your own decision, we'd like to expand your horizons a little. Our goal in sharing other weaning practices is not to convince you to follow them but to give you a broader perspective on your options. We find it sad that some women wean before they feel ready because others convince them that they are being "selfish" or harming their child by breastfeeding past a certain age. As you will see, the age that our culture considers normal for weaning is at the very early end of the human spectrum. We hope that knowing this will give you more freedom to make your own decisions.

OTHER TIMES AND PLACES

If human societies were viewed as a whole, the average age of weaning would be between two and four years of age. Until the twentieth century, children in both China and Japan breastfed until ages four or five. In 1967, famed anthropologist Margaret Mead and early breastfeeding researcher Niles Newton published an article describing the weaning practices of sixty-four traditional cultures. Among all these cultures, only one routinely weaned children as young as six months (Mead and Newton 1967).

History tells us that breastfeeding for years was common practice in most times and places. The Koran recommends breastfeeding until age two, and the custom of the Egyptian pharaohs in Moses's time was to breastfeed for three years. Even in England and the United States, historical writings tell us that not so long ago, two to four years of breastfeeding was typical. In 1725, authors of child-care texts clearly disapproved of four-year-olds breastfeeding, which implies there were more than a few of them around. By 1850, breastfeeding for eleven months was recommended and breastfeeding for two years was criticized. Historically, weaning was considered a dangerous time. In the old West, tombstones of children often listed "weaning death" as the cause (Bumgarner 2000).

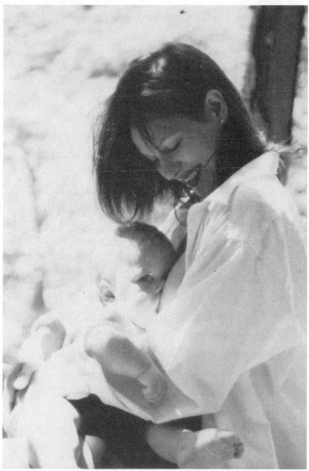

Breastfeeding provides comfort and emotional security to older babies as they venture into the wider world. (©2005 Mary Jane Chase, RNC, MN, CCE, IBCLC, used with permission)

IS THERE A HUMAN NORM?

In the 1995 book, *Breastfeeding: Biocultural Perspectives*, coeditor Katherine Dettwyler, a cultural anthropologist, attempts to define a biological "human norm" for age of weaning, apart from the influence of culture. To do this, she applied the following criteria, which biologists use to estimate the natural weaning age of other mammals:

- age at which birth weight is tripled or quadrupled (in humans, two to three years)

- age at which offspring reach one-third of adult weight (in humans, four to seven years)

- age of eruption of permanent teeth (in humans, five-and-a-half to six years of age, the same age at which our immune systems become fully developed)

- relationship to length of pregnancy (chimpanzees, our nearest relative, breastfeed for six times the length of their pregnancy, which for humans would be four-and-a-half years)

By applying these criteria to humans, she concluded that the natural age of weaning, or the human norm, is between two-and-a-half and seven years (Dettwyler 1995).

Are we suggesting that you should breastfeed this long? Not at all. We simply want you to know that if you decide to breastfeed longer than most people you know, it is not harmful to either you or your child. On the contrary, as former U.S. Surgeon General Antonia Novello said, "It's the lucky baby, I feel, who continues to nurse until he's two" (Novello 1990, 5).

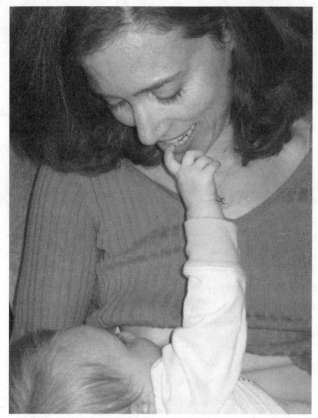

As baby grows, breastfeeding becomes more about giving and receiving love than about the milk. (©2010 Mary Jane Chase, RNC, MN, CCE, IBCLC, used with permission)

Reasons to Wean

There are many reasons women give for weaning, and some of these reasons are entirely justified, while others deserve deeper thought.

REASONS TO THINK TWICE ABOUT WEANING

You may want to think twice if weaning will not accomplish your intended goal or if critical information is missing. The following are some of the reasons women wean unnecessarily.

An unsolved breastfeeding problem for which you haven't sought expert help. A mother in the midst of a breastfeeding crisis often genuinely believes that her situation is hopeless. She may feel as if she has tried everything, even if she hasn't yet sought help from a lactation professional. If you find yourself in this situation, know that a board-certified lactation consultant can most likely offer new strategies you haven't tried. When you have a breastfeeding problem, you need someone both skilled and objective who can help you sort out what is happening and work with you to come up with a solution. Remember, babies are hardwired to breastfeed, and almost all problems are fixable. Don't give up before you've worked with an expert. As we said in the chapters 5 and 6, the most common reason given for premature weaning is "worries about milk production," which are most often due to simple confusion about what's normal.

You're returning to work. Many mothers manage working and breastfeeding very successfully. Lactation consultant Robyn Roche-Paull writes that even women in active-duty military service can still manage to at least partially breastfeed (for more on that, see her site www.breastfeedingincombatboots.com; Roche-Paull 2010). Even if you can't express your milk at work, you can still breastfeed when you're home. Some breastfeeding is always better than none. (See "Partial Weaning," later in this chapter, on how to do this. We also provide some specific strategies for working and breastfeeding in chapter 9.)

One medical opinion. As we'll describe in more detail in chapter 8, we live in a strange world where most health care professionals have had little to no breastfeeding training or education. This isn't just our opinion. In a survey of 3,115 residents and 1,920 practicing physicians in pediatrics, family practice, and obstetrics, a substantial percentage of respondents gave incorrect responses when asked specific questions about breastfeeding management and seemed unaware of the negative health outcomes of nonhuman milks (Freed, Clark, Lohr, et al. 1995; Freed, Clark, Sorenson, et al. 1995).

Yet this lack of knowledge and training doesn't seem to prevent the average physician from giving advice. (One amazing "medical reason" for weaning we've heard lately is, "Your baby is allergic to your milk," which is physically impossible.) There are obviously some exceptions to this. We both know physicians who are not only knowledgeable but are leaders in the field. However, if a health care provider recommends weaning, it's time to get a second opinion. You may want to start by contacting a local lactation consultant or a mother-to-mother breast-feeding counselor for the name of breastfeeding-savvy health care professionals in your area.

Along these lines, we get many calls from breastfeeding mothers concerned about medications. We'll cover this in more detail in chapter 9. But know now that most drugs are compatible with breastfeeding. Furthermore, in most cases the risks of giving formula are greater than the risks of taking the drug and continuing to breastfeed. But if you are prescribed one of the rare drugs that is incompatible with breastfeeding, you may still have options. The doctor may be able to substitute another drug. Even if not, you have the option of temporarily weaning, continuing to express your milk, and returning to breastfeeding later.

Mother or baby is ill or hospitalized. This is usually the worst time to wean, as an ill baby will almost always recover faster on human milk. And the last thing an ill or injured mother needs is the pain and health risks of an abrupt weaning (see "Risks to You of Abrupt Weaning" at the end of this chapter).

Pregnancy. Some women choose to wean during pregnancy, but you don't have to. There is no evidence that breastfeeding is harmful in any way to the unborn baby. The only caution we would give is if you are at risk for preterm birth. The mild uterine contractions that breastfeeding can cause may be of concern if there is a risk of going into labor early. If this is the case, you've probably also been told to abstain from sex until after delivery as well.

Baby has teeth. In most places, babies breastfeed long past the age of teething. If biting is a problem for you and your baby, see chapter 10 on ways to stop the biting without weaning.

Baby's on strike. If your baby "weans herself" before one year, chances are it is not a natural weaning but a "nursing strike." If this happens to you, see chapter 10 for ways to get your baby back to breastfeeding.

So baby will sleep better. Despite popular belief, research has found that starting solids doesn't help babies sleep better or longer (see

"Solids and sleep" later in this chapter). In fact, several recent studies have found that mothers who exclusively breastfeed actually get more sleep than mothers who formula feed or who both breast- and bottle-feed (Doan et al. 2007; Gay, Lee, and Lee 2004).

To encourage independence. There is no evidence weaning will do this. In fact, you might find that an abruptly weaned baby becomes more clingy and dependent.

To make your life easier. We're all for making mothers' lives easier. But weaning is no guarantee of this. In fact, you might find that life gets more challenging once you wean your baby. Once weaned, if your child wakes at night, you now have to get out of bed to settle her down. She is likely to get sick more often. And you will lose the calming and comforting mothering tool of breastfeeding. We also know a few mothers who weaned only to find that their babies could not tolerate any of the formulas available and that they had to go back to breast-feeding. We don't want you to be disappointed, or worse, find that your life becomes more difficult. Think carefully before weaning for this reason.

YOUR TIME TO WEAN HAS COME

When it's time to wean, be sure you have all the facts, know all your options, and you (or your baby) make the decision to wean. The following reasons indicate your time may have come.

You're ready. You've met your goals or have decided to wean based on your own unique considerations. Or you've simply decided the time is right.

Your child's ready. As Law 7 says, even if you do nothing to wean your child, all children will eventually wean naturally (see "Natural Weaning" later in this chapter), sometimes even before their mothers are ready to wean. Natural weaning can happen as young as twelve months.

There's a confirmed medical issue. By "confirmed" we mean that you've gotten a second opinion as well as spoken to a lactation con-sultant. Many mothers wean unnecessarily on the recommendation of a health care provider who later proves to be wrong. We have worked with mothers who were told to wean so they could get a mammogram, which is completely unnecessary. Two medically valid reasons to wean involving a mother's health include chemotherapy for cancer or radioactive therapy for thyroid problems.

OTHER REASONS TO WEAN

Some reasons to wean can be trickier to negotiate and deserve some extra thought.

Feeling overwhelmed with breastfeeding. If this is your reason, we hope you have sought skilled breastfeeding help. Often there are ways to make breastfeeding easier. But there are some mothers (for example, those who were sexually abused in childhood) for whom breastfeeding can feel overwhelming even when it's going well. If you do feel overwhelmed, you still have options. Women who have difficulty with the close body contact of breastfeeding sometimes pump their milk and give it to their baby by bottle. Some do a partial weaning, eliminating some regular breastfeedings until they feel more at ease. Some breastfeeding is always better than none. See the section "Past Sexual Abuse or Sexual Assault" in chapter 11 for more suggestions.

Social or family pressures. Some women find themselves in a family or an environment in which breastfeeding is frowned upon. It takes a strong person to breastfeed in spite of an unsupportive partner, family, or social circle. If this is your problem, consider finding the support you need elsewhere. In one study, mother-to-mother support was essential to maintaining breastfeeding when mothers were feeling pressured to wean. Family members and strangers were the two groups of people most likely to be critical of mothers who breastfed for longer than six months (Kendall-Tackett and Sugarman 1995). Many mothers attend weekly mothers' meetings at a hospital, monthly mother-to-mother breastfeeding groups (for example, La Leche League, Nursing Mothers Counsel, Australian Breastfeeding Association), or both, as an antidote to the negativity they face in the wider world. Online groups can also be an important source of support, especially for mothers who don't have access to breastfeeding groups in their communities. Meeting with other like-minded women—even once a month—can make a tremendous difference. You might also check to see if there are any Breastfeeding or Baby Cafes where you can drop in and talk with other women. For many mothers, that type of breastfeeding support fits in better with their lifestyles.

What Mothers Say About Weaning

Your feelings are an important part of the weaning equation. If you are considering weaning because you find breastfeeding stressful, it may help to know what mothers with the benefit of hindsight say about weaning. In one 1987 study, Cosby Rogers and his colleagues asked women their feelings about weaning, well after the fact, and found that 65 percent who weaned their babies at three months or younger had regrets. More than 50 percent of those who weaned at four to six months wished they had breastfed longer (Rogers, Morris, and Taper 1987). Norma Jane Bumgarner, author of *Mothering Your Nursing Toddler* (2000), a book for those who breastfeed past one year, noted after reading letters from hundreds of mothers, that those who most consistently described feelings of loss and regret after weaning were those who weaned before two years.

> When nursing continues past two or three years, mothers much less frequently describe weaning in the same mixed terms. It seems that a time comes in the growth of the mother-child relationship when it is easier for both to move on and leave baby things behind (Bumgarner 2000, 288).

If you are considering weaning before you had intended to because of mixed or negative feelings, you owe it to both your baby and yourself to talk to a breastfeeding professional to see if there is a solution or adjustment that would help you feel better about continuing.

Weaning Basics

When your time comes to wean, remember Law 7: *Children wean naturally.* We hope that knowing this law, along with the following information, will help you navigate this inevitable transition comfortably and happily.

Why Gradual Weaning Is Better

Ideally, weaning should always be done gradually. Unfortunately, gradual weaning runs counter to the most commonly given advice, which is to stop breastfeeding abruptly, bind the breasts, and wait for the pain to subside. This is a barbaric approach that is unnecessarily painful and risky.

To appreciate why, consider the alternative. If weaning is gradual enough, you will never feel pain or discomfort. You will also avoid health risks, which include a painful complication that could require hospitalization and surgery (see "Risks to You of Abrupt Weaning" later in this chapter). For your baby, a gradual weaning will give you the time to make sure she tolerates well whatever formula or other food you substitute before your milk is gone. A gradual weaning also allows you to give your baby more focused attention and comforting skin-to-skin contact to make the emotional adjustment easier for her. Since breastfeeding is a part of your close relationship, you want your baby to know that you are not withdrawing your love along with your breasts.

Approaches to Weaning

As we said at the beginning, your approach to weaning makes all the difference. Let's take a closer look at some of your choices and how they work.

REDUCING MILK PRODUCTION COMFORTABLY

As you wean, your goal is to reduce your milk production gradually and comfortably. To do this, let's apply what we learned in chapter 6 in reverse. As we explained, milk production is determined by how many times per day—and how well—milk is drained from the breasts, either by a baby or by pumping. So to decrease your milk production gradually, you can do one or both of the following:

- Gradually decrease the amount of milk drained from the breasts each time.

- Gradually decrease the number of times per day the breasts are drained.

However, as with many things in life, the devil is in the details. The following sections describe different approaches to weaning and how these principles apply.

NATURAL WEANING

Let's start with the approach that most U.S. mothers seem to know the least about, but when considered within the big picture of human history, may be the most commonly used. This approach is to allow your baby to outgrow breastfeeding, otherwise known as *natural weaning*.

Why some choose natural weaning. Even in the United States, where 77 percent of babies are weaned by one year, some mothers choose natural weaning. Some choose it because it feels right to them. Others choose it because it allows their children to grow at their own pace and wean according to their own inner timetable. Still others choose natural weaning because it requires the least work.

Although the uninitiated sometimes assume that breastfeeding past one year is an act of martyrdom, mothers report that in many ways breastfeeding a toddler makes their lives easier. The relaxing breastfeeding hormones help mothers keep their cool, even under duress. And as a mothering tool, breastfeeding continues to make naptimes and bedtimes blissfully easy as well as ending tantrums in the blink of an eye.

Natural weaning is usually gradual, although an occasional toddler may naturally wean earlier and more abruptly than her mother expects. More commonly, though, your milk production reduces slowly and comfortably, without any thought or effort, as your child's attention becomes more focused on the world around her and less on you. Another plus of natural weaning is that you never have to deal with an unhappy child resisting your efforts to wean or the hassle of weaning from the bottle later. As one mother said, "I wouldn't think of limiting or ending the breastfeeding relationship any more than I would think of limiting or ending my love for my children. Gradual weaning allowed us both to grow into other ways of expressing our love" (Kendall-Tackett and Sugarman 1995, 181). Many women who wean naturally report that the process was so gradual that they are not even sure when their child's last breastfeeding happened.

At what age do children naturally wean? Many mothers worry that if they don't take the lead in weaning that their child will breastfeed "forever." In reality, all children outgrow breastfeeding. How long does it take? It varies from child to child, like the age a child learns to walk and talk, or gets her first tooth. One child may wean at one or two years while another may be avidly breastfeeding at three. A child with a strong sucking urge, an intense need for closeness, or an unrecognized allergy or other physical problem may breastfeed longer than others.

Social challenges. As we described earlier, one study found that for many U.S. mothers, the biggest challenge of natural weaning is coping with others' opinions, and the older the child, the more challenging this becomes. Yet, in spite of this, the mothers in the study felt that the positives outweighed the negatives (Kendall-Tackett and Sugarman 1995).

One way to handle social challenges is to keep breastfeeding private. This is an option because an older child does not usually breastfeed as often as a young baby. Some tried-and-true strategies for avoiding breastfeeding in a less-than-friendly environment include the following:

- setting limits on where and when your child can breastfeed

- bringing snacks, drinks, toys, and/or books to distract your child when you go out

- choosing a "code word" for breastfeeding that won't be obvious to others

- finding private places to breastfeed outside the home, such as fitting rooms or "mothers' lounges" at the mall

- carefully choosing your clothing (two-piece outfits are best; cover-ups like ponchos or shawls can help, too)

The importance of support. Mothers who breastfeed longer than their cultural norm enjoy the experience more if they have support. Mother-to-mother breastfeeding groups like La Leche League, Nursing Mothers Counsel, and the Australian Breastfeeding Association are great places to meet others who value breastfeeding over a wide range of ages.

PLANNED WEANING AFTER ONE YEAR

Let's say your goal is to breastfeed for one or two years, but you prefer to wean before your child outgrows breastfeeding. If so, this section is for you.

Even though the child one year or older may have strong preferences about breastfeeding—as she will about all aspects of her daily routine—you can still make weaning a gradual and positive experience. To accomplish this, first allow plenty of time. It may take several weeks to wean, depending on how many times a day she has been breastfeeding. You also need to consider her temperament and opinions, and factor them into your strategies. Think about alternatives that she might consider to be even better than breastfeeding, because, as author and pediatrician Dr. William Sears says, "A wise baby who enjoys a happy nursing relationship is not likely to give it up willingly unless some other form of emotional nourishment is provided that is equally attractive or at least interestingly different" (cited in Mohrbacher 1995, 41). The following strategies are among your many options.

Don't offer, don't refuse. Breastfeed when she asks but otherwise don't offer. When used with other strategies, this one can speed up the process.

Offer regular meals, snacks, and drinks. Minimize her hunger and thirst with alternatives to breastfeeding, and offer her age-appropriate fun activities to avoid breastfeeding out of boredom.

Change daily routines. Think about the times and places she asks to breastfeed and how to change your routine so she will be reminded less often. For example, if she usually asks to breastfeed when you sit in a certain chair, avoid that chair.

Get your partner involved. If she usually breastfeeds first thing in the morning, ask your partner to get her up and give her breakfast. Your partner can also help her get back to sleep when she wakes at night and plan special daytime outings for her to distract her from her usual routine.

Anticipate and offer substitutes and distractions. Be sure to offer substitutes before she asks to breastfeed, because once she's asked, she will likely feel rejected and upset if a substitute is offered. As an example, right before a usual breastfeeding time, offer a special snack and drink and then take her to a favorite place, such as a playground, as a distraction. Some children breastfeed more often at home with nothing to do and less when out and distracted. For this type of child, spend as much of the day as possible out of the house. Other children breastfeed more often when in new surroundings. For a child like this, stay home more and keep distractions to a minimum.

Postpone. This works for a child who breastfeeds at irregular times and places and is old enough to accept waiting. If postponing leaves your child feeling as though you are keeping her at arm's length, she may become even more determined to breastfeed. If so, use other strategies.

Shorten the length of breastfeedings. This is most effective with children older than two and is a good beginning to the weaning process.

Bargaining. This one can work well with the older child. A child who is close to outgrowing breastfeeding may give up breastfeeding earlier by mutual agreement. But most children younger than three do not have the maturity and perspective to understand the meaning of a promise.

Adjust your plan based on your child's reactions and preferences. Pick and choose among these strategies based on your child's reactions. One child may be unhappy with postponing but do well with distraction and substitution. Also, certain breastfeedings may be more important to your child than others. If so, continue those until the end and allow your child to give them up last. If she clings to these breastfeedings, you can continue with them for a while. Often the bedtime breastfeeding is a favorite.

Be flexible. When unusual situations arise, avoid sticking rigidly to your weaning strategies. If your child is ill, she may want to breastfeed more often for comfort. You can go back to weaning after she's feeling better.

When to slow down. Even at the same age, some children will be more ready to wean than others. If your child becomes upset and cries or insists upon breastfeeding even when you try to distract or comfort her in others ways, this may mean that weaning is going too fast for her or that different strategies would be better. Other signs that weaning may be moving too fast are changes or regressions in behavior, such as stuttering, night-waking, an increase in clinginess, a new or increased fear of separation, biting (if she has never bitten before), stomach upsets, and constipation.

Make weaning a positive experience for your child by paying attention to your own inner voice and being sensitive to your child's cues.

PLANNED WEANING OF A YOUNGER BABY

When weaning a child younger than one year, the nutritional aspects of breastfeeding need to be considered first. So before beginning to wean, consult your baby's health care provider for recommendations for human milk substitutes. The feeding method you choose will depend upon your baby's age. If she is close to a year old and drinking well from a cup, you may be able to forego the bottle entirely and go directly to a cup, which avoids the need to wean again from a bottle later.

The practical details of weaning. If she is much younger than twelve months, you'll need to substitute some type of formula for breastfeeding, as regular cow's milk is not recommended until after one year. Here's how to wean step by step at this stage:

1. Make note of the times you usually breastfeed.

2. Pick one daily breastfeeding (except the first morning breast-feeding; leave that for last) and substitute formula by bottle (or cup, for the older baby).

3. Give your body at least two to three days to adjust before dropping another breastfeeding so that your milk production has time to decrease comfortably and gradually.

4. If at any time your breasts feel full, express just enough milk to feel comfortable (pump just to comfort—no longer) or allow the baby to breastfeed for a short time. There are health risks to allowing your breasts to get or stay uncomfortably full. Pay attention to your body's cues, expressing milk to comfort whenever needed.

Following this plan, it usually takes about two to three weeks to go from exclusive breastfeeding to a complete weaning.

When you're down to breastfeeding just once or twice a day, if there is no rush to wean completely, you can continue these breastfeedings for as long as you like. Your breasts will continue to produce enough milk as long as your baby breastfeeds. Remember, some breastfeeding is always better than none.

The importance of reassurance. A gradual weaning like this gives you time to make sure your baby is adjusting well to the change and to give her extra focused and loving attention as a substitute for the closeness you shared while breastfeeding.

Other outlets for sucking. Because babies come hardwired with a strong need to suck until the natural age of weaning, they may find another outlet, such as thumbsucking, during or after weaning. If you prefer that your baby use a bottle or pacifier, you can offer one of these instead.

PARTIAL WEANING

This can be an alternative to total weaning for the mother who finds the body contact of breastfeeding difficult or some other aspect of breastfeeding either impractical or overwhelming. It can also be a compromise for the mother returning to work who doesn't plan to express her milk while away from her baby. A partial weaning can allow her to continue breastfeeding when she's home and yet bring her milk production down to the point where she doesn't have to pump at work.

To do a partial weaning, follow the step-by-step instructions in "The practical details of weaning," above, to decrease your number of breastfeedings until your milk production adjusts gradually downward. Once you have reached the point that your breasts do not get uncomfortably full for the length of time you're away from your baby, you can continue with that number of breastfeedings. Once there, you can continue breastfeeding at this level for as long as you like.

ABRUPT WEANING

Although this is the least desirable of your options, abrupt weaning is sometimes necessary in cases of tragedy (the death of a baby) or a medical emergency. If it becomes necessary, consider your options, get a second opinion, and talk to a lactation consultant. Many times there are alternatives to weaning you may be unaware of. If an abrupt weaning is unavoidable

- wear a firm bra for support (one size larger than usual so it does not get too tight);

- reduce your salt intake but not your fluids;

- express milk as needed to stay comfortable.

To wean quickly, use an effective breast pump (such as a rental pump) to make the process as gradual and comfortable as possible. As your milk production decreases, the need to express milk also decreases. **Remember**: Do not wait to express milk until you are overly full or in pain. There are health risks to unrelieved breast fullness. (See "Risks to You of Abrupt Weaning" at the end of this chapter.)

Attend to your baby's emotional needs. An abrupt weaning is the most stressful option for you and your baby. No matter what her age, breastfeeding is part of her close relationship with you. Keep this in mind and be sure baby gets lots of focused attention and skin-to-skin contact to reassure her that you have not withdrawn your love. If you are not available, be sure your baby has someone else to hold and comfort her.

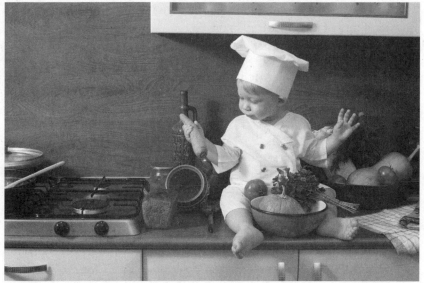

Signs of readiness for solid foods include the ability to sit up and pick up food.

The Role of Solid Foods

Depending on the age of your child, the introduction of solid foods may play a significant role in the weaning process. As we described at the beginning of this chapter, outside the United States "weaning" is often defined as the introduction of solids.

Solids and Milk Production

An important point to know is that when solid foods are introduced, they do not increase a baby's overall intake. Solids take the place of your milk or formula in your baby's diet. If you are exclusively breastfeeding, this changes the equation that determines your milk production. In chapter 6, we described how milk production is based on the number of times per day your breasts are drained and how well they are drained. As your baby takes more solids, she takes less milk.

This is why your timing and strategy for giving solid foods can affect your long-term breastfeeding goals.

When to Start Solids

A generation ago, mothers were encouraged to give their babies solids within the first six weeks. But as the practice of early solids was studied, researchers found serious drawbacks for both mothers and babies, and this practice was abandoned. As we mentioned in chapter 6, the still-common recommendation of starting solid foods at four to six months is now being revised. In 2001, the World Health Organization's panel of experts examined the available research on the ideal age for starting solids and concluded that waiting to start solids for a full six months results in better health outcomes for mothers and babies (WHO 2001). Because a younger baby's digestive system is not yet mature enough to handle solid foods well, babies who start solids before six months are at higher risk for the following:

- allergies

- ear infections

- digestive problems

When solids are given too early, a more age-appropriate food is being replaced with a food that your baby cannot yet fully digest. But because solid foods fill her up and make her less interested in breast-feeding, the earlier solids are started, the greater the risk that a mother's milk production will be reduced before mother or baby is ready to wean.

You may not want to delay solids for too long either. Several recent studies have found that delaying solids beyond six months can also increase the risk of illnesses such as celiac disease or type 1 diabetes (Agostoni et al. 2008).

BABY'S SIGNS OF READINESS

On a practical level, giving solids to babies younger than six months is difficult because babies are born with a tongue-thrust reflex; this causes your baby to push out with her tongue anything that goes into her mouth. This tongue thrusting, which is usually outgrown between four and six months, often makes feeding a young baby solids an exercise in frustration.

What we're beginning to understand is that physical readiness for solids coincides with your baby's ability to feed herself, which makes good, logical sense. Your baby is most likely ready for solids when she reaches this level of maturity and you see the following signs of readiness:

- She can sit up alone.

- She can pick up food and put it in her mouth.

- Her tongue-thrust reflex has disappeared.

- She shows an interest in eating other foods.

This last point is crucial, as experience has shown that babies who are at risk for allergies tend to refuse solids until they are a little older, possibly in an effort to protect their sensitive digestive systems. So if a baby does not want solids exactly at six months, it is best to continue to offer them about once a week but to let your baby take the lead.

SIGNS TO IGNORE

The following are *not* indicators of a baby's readiness for solids:

- Baby reaches a certain weight (despite what commercial baby food companies say).

- Baby is not sleeping well at night (see "Solids and sleep" on this, later in this chapter).

How to Start Solids

Keep in mind that between six months and nine months or so, your baby needs your milk more than she needs solid foods. This means that the amount of solid foods she takes is less important than the practice she's getting. Think of this as a time when she learns to eat solids before they really matter to her nutritionally.

A BABY-LED APPROACH TO SOLIDS

In their book *Baby-led Weaning*, British midwife Gill Rapley and writer Tracey Murkett describe how a baby's introduction to solids can be baby-led (Rapley and Murkett 2008). When babies feed themselves, rather than being fed, they control how much they eat, stopping when they are full. In the process, they learn to recognize fullness, which will help them develop healthy eating habits.

Start with foods babies can pick up by themselves. Initially, more of the food will end up on the floor or on your baby's face and hands than in your baby's stomach. But that's okay because most of your baby's nutrition is coming from your milk.

During this process, your baby will gnaw and play with her food and also actually eat some. This can be messy, so use bibs, undress baby to a diaper, bathe after feedings, and/or put plastic down around baby's chair. Let your baby experience food with all her senses and decide how much food she wants to eat.

There is no need to puree foods and feed the baby. And there is no need for special baby food. Your baby can share what your family eats, and you can all eat at the same time, which makes meal times a lot more pleasant for everyone (Rapley and Murkett 2008).

GETTING STARTED

Rapley and Murkett also recommend a few steps to take before your baby begins eating. First, wash your baby's hands since she will be eating with her hands and handling her food. Second, your baby should be sitting upright, either in a high chair or on your lap. Never offer solid foods to your baby if you are not right there with her. Third, prepare for a mess.

Types of first foods. Babies can eat many types of regular foods. The foods given to babies when they start solids vary around the world depending on the locale, the culture, the season, and the foods available. When deciding on a food for your baby, keep in mind that fresh foods are more nutritious than processed foods. Some finger foods that Rapley and Murkett (2008) recommend include the following:

- steamed whole vegetables, such as green beans, snap peas, or baby sweet corn

- steamed cauliflower or broccoli florets (these are great because they have built-in "handles")

- steamed or roasted vegetable sticks such as sweet potato, carrot, or zucchini

- thin strips of meat, such as chicken, beef, or pork. These can be served warm or cold.

- pasta

- strips of bread

- fruit, either whole or in sticks (apple, pear, mango, peach, banana)

Solids to avoid for one year. Foods best avoided until a baby is one year old include cow's milk, egg whites, peanuts, citrus fruits, shellfish, honey (due to botulism spores), and any food of a size and shape that might block baby's windpipe, such as hot dogs and raw carrots (wait until baby is three).

Signs of food sensitivity. The following are signs a baby is reacting badly to a food:

- hives, diaper rash, or eczema

- runny nose or congestion

- wheezing

- red, itchy eyes

- ear infection

- fussiness

- digestive problems—constipation, vomiting, diarrhea

If you see any of these signs, eliminate that food and try it again the next week. If baby reacts again, avoid that food for several months.

Solids to avoid in allergic families. It used to be recommended that some foods be delayed for one year in families with a history of allergies. These foods included wheat, corn, pork, fish, tomatoes, onions, cabbage, berries, nuts, and spices. However, evidence has recently come to light indicating that avoiding these foods for one year does not prevent allergy, and so this is no longer recommended (Greer, Sicherer, and Burks 2008).

Solids and sleep. Many parents are anxious to start solid foods because they've heard that solids will help their babies sleep better. However, two studies that monitored babies' sleep habits found no correlation between solid foods and sleep (Macknin, Medendorp, and Maier 1989; Keane et al. 1988). The same number of babies slept through the night whether they hadn't yet started solids or had been given rice cereal right before bed. In their 1989 study, Michael Macknin and his colleagues concluded that "...infants' ability to sleep through the night is a developmental and adaptive process that occurs regardless of the timing of introduction of cereal" (Macknin, Medendorp, and Maier 1989, 1,068).

When the System Breaks Down

Throughout this chapter we have alluded to the risks of abrupt weaning. Now it's time to get more specific. If you ever find yourself in a situation in which abrupt weaning is recommended, as we've said, it is wise to get a second opinion and talk to a lactation consultant, because other options can usually be found.

Risks of Abrupt Weaning

Unfortunately, when a mother asks how to wean, abrupt weaning is often the first and only approach she is given. As mentioned, many health care providers tell mothers to simply stop breastfeeding, bind their breasts, and wait until the pain subsides. (That's easy for them to say!) This is an unnecessarily stressful and risky way to wean. Now let's examine why.

RISKS TO YOU OF ABRUPT WEANING

The physical risks to you of a sudden weaning are the most obvious and are reason enough to take a gradual approach.

Pain. When a mother stops breastfeeding suddenly, her breasts continue making milk. When the milk is not removed, her breasts become full, fuller, overly full, and then painfully engorged. Some women describe the pain they've suffered with abrupt weaning as the worst pain they've ever experienced. We've received frantic calls from weaning mothers in pain who ask what to do to relieve it. "Breastfeed or pump" is our usual reply. There's no reason in the world to endure this pain when weaning can be done comfortably and gradually.

Mastitis. Unrelieved breast fullness is one cause of *mastitis*, which is an inflammation of the breasts. Mastitis can be mild or severe and covers a spectrum of symptoms.

Mild mastitis, or *plugged ducts*, causes sore, lumpy areas in the breast. They are usually easily treated, but if the milk is not removed well and often, it can progress to a more severe form of mastitis, in which the sore areas become red and hot and the mother develops a fever and flu-like symptoms. The best treatment for mastitis is frequent breast drainage, either by breastfeeding (which is preferred) or by breast pumping, along with warm compresses and rest. But if a mother with mastitis is weaning (not recommended!) and she does not drain the milk from her breasts often, the condition can worsen. If her breast fullness is unrelieved and her mastitis with fever is not treated quickly with the right antibiotics, the condition can progress into its most severe form: breast abscess. For more details on mastitis treatments, see chapter 10.

Breast abscess. A breast abscess is a pus-filled cyst in the breast. When a mother develops this complication, which happens in 5–11 percent of women with infectious mastitis who receive incorrect or delayed treatment, she may need to be hospitalized and have the abscess drained surgically. **Note:** Due to this risk, weaning is never recommended during mastitis. See chapter 10 for more information on mastitis.

Emotional distress. Women who have been forced to wean before they are ready often speak of the sadness and despair they felt. They grieve the loss of breastfeeding and its special closeness.

RISKS TO YOUR BABY OF ABRUPT WEANING

When breastfeeding is withdrawn suddenly, a baby can also have physical and emotional reactions.

Reactions to alternative foods. A baby who is allergic or sensitive to nonhuman milks or other foods may have a strong physical reaction when breastfeeding is withdrawn suddenly and her system is flooded with triggering foods (for specifics, see the possible reactions to solids listed in "Signs of food sensitivity," above). A gradual weaning allows a mother to determine her baby's tolerance of other foods before moving forward. It also gives her time to reconsider, if her baby doesn't handle the alternatives well. We've both worked with mothers who have completely stopped breastfeeding only to need to start again because their babies could not tolerate any other foods.

Emotional distress. Because breastfeeding is a source of comfort and closeness as well as food, an abrupt weaning is emotionally stressful to your baby. If you have no choice but to wean abruptly, make every effort to give your baby lots of reassurance, focused attention, and skin-to-skin contact.

Summary

Weaning need not be a painful process for you or your baby. For your and baby's sake, avoid abrupt weaning if at all possible. You can choose to allow your child to wean naturally. Or, if you choose to take the lead, going slowly will help. You avoid the possible physical and emotional complications that can occur, and you give yourself time to evaluate how well your baby is adapting to weaning. By waiting until your child is ready or by easing off breastfeeding gradually and expressing your love in other ways, weaning can be a joyful celebration of your child's coming of age, or at the very least, a positive experience for both of you.

CHAPTER 8

What Interferes
with the Laws

In the first seven chapters, we described how simple breastfeeding can be and how important it is to the health of mothers and babies. If what we say is true, then you might wonder how our culture has managed to stray so far from breastfeeding as the biological norm for you and your baby. That's the focus of this chapter. To answer this question, we must take you on a brief excursion through history. Understanding how we got to this point is important since much of the bad breast-feeding advice you will receive stems from specific historical and cultural movements and related beliefs. If you know where various ideas came from, you'll be in a much better position to evaluate them and decide whether they will work for you and your family. Here we go.

The Role of History and Culture

To understand where we are now, we need to go back about 150 to 200 years ago to when the Industrial Revolution was in full swing. Starting in the 1830s, a wider variety of mass-produced products became available and people's standards of living began to rise. Innovation was equated with improvement in everyday comfort. Products that we all now take for granted, like reliable sources of heat and light and indoor plumbing, were, for the first time, widely available to ordinary people. The amount of change that families experienced during this time was unprecedented. It seemed like every day brought a new innovation that made problems that people had dealt with for millennia suddenly disappear. The old ways of doing things suddenly seemed out of place in the new technological age.

Science was also making significant advances, most notably in the battle against disease. Problems that had terrorized people for thousands of years were overcome. There was the advent of anesthesia (which allowed doctors to operate without killing their patients from shock), effective pain relief, and the germ theory of infection. Mortality rates dropped. It was a heady time. Science seemed to hold the promise of eradicating all human misery, while many traditional methods of health and healing were seen as out of step.

The Rise of Scientific Mothering

It wasn't long before the lens of science and technology was turned upon mothers and babies. Soon scientists, in the thrall of American

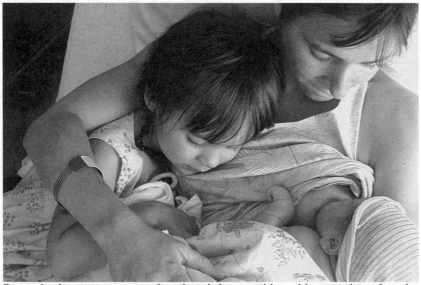

Breastfeeding gives you a free hand for an older sibling and is also the best, most natural way to teach breastfeeding norms to the next generation. (©Marilyn Nolt, used with permission)

behaviorism, pronounced that the only proper way to raise a baby was with "scientific mothering." *Behaviorism* was an important theory in the social sciences for a significant part of the twentieth century. Its emphasis was on how the environment shaped people's and animals' responses through rewards and punishments. Proponents of this theory implied, or explicitly stated, that parents could get the kind of children they wanted via reinforcements and punishments. For example, if you want children who cry less often, don't respond to them (i.e., reinforce them) when they cry. Parenting manuals in which male experts could share with mothers the "latest techniques" first became really popular during the early part of the twentieth century. Mothers were advised not to spoil their babies with affection, to provide them with a clean and sterile environment, and to use a strict schedule for everything from eating to sleeping to toilet training.

FEEDING BY THE CLOCK

One of the beliefs that grew out of the scientific-mothering approach was that babies should be fed at predetermined intervals. The clock, rather than a baby's sense of hunger, should determine when he should be fed next. We are still dealing with the impact of this mistaken belief today.

You can see how breastfeeding would be unappealing to those who adopted this regularized and "scientific" approach to raising children. Breastfeeding is more intuitive, relying upon mothers' being able to read their babies' cues. Mothers and babies determine when the baby has had enough, rather than outside experts. The whole process of breastfeeding seemed sloppy and messy and completely unscientific.

NONHUMAN MILKS

It was against this backdrop that manufactured baby milks first became widely commercially available and gained broad acceptance. In this era of scientific mothering, these products—called "formula" in reference to their scientific origins—were actually touted as being better for babies than their mothers' milk.

Prior to this time, people had experimented with all manner of substitutes for human milk, and, unfortunately, in most places many babies died as a result. Some examples of food given to babies were beer, "sops" (bread soaked in milk or water), and gruel (cereal). It's a wonder that any survived this kind of regimen. Babies of wealthy families were also often put out to *wet-nurse* with other women who were hired to breastfeed the babies. Even with breastfeeding, many of these babies died—perhaps due to neglect by wet nurses who were caring for too many babies at once (it was said that wet nurses were "limited" to six babies at a time) or because wet nurses were impoverished themselves and could not provide proper care.

Around the same time that nonhuman baby milks became commercially available, pediatrics, a new medical specialty, came into existence. Mothers were told that rather than using family-practice doctors, as before, they should take their babies to the new "baby doctors," because they were trained to create formulas to meet each baby's individual needs. (For more information on the history of this era and the ties between pediatrics and the formula industry, see the Resources section for *The Politics of Breastfeeding: Why Breasts Are Bad for Business* by Gabrielle Palmer.) Formula also appealed to a science-enamored generation because it was easy to tell just how much milk a baby took at each feeding. Therefore, feeding could be regulated and monitored in a precise way. It sounded like a great system—except for the fact that babies were dying.

THE PRICE OF PROGRESS

As early as the 1920s, researchers found that babies fed with nonhuman milks died at a rate that was three to six times higher than their breastfed counterparts (Woodbury 1925). And that was in the United States. The picture was far bleaker in the developing world, and it still is today.

UNETHICAL MARKETING PRACTICES

As the decades passed and their products became widely used in developed countries like the United States, formula companies realized that developing nations were also a potentially lucrative market. In a shameful chapter in the history of this industry, women were hired to dress like nurses and offer free samples of formula to mothers—

just enough so that their milk production would decrease or disappear. Then women thought they had no choice but to continue to buy formula, even when they couldn't afford it and even when they had to mix it with contaminated water. The irresponsibility of these multinational corporations led to worldwide boycotts of their products. The death rate was staggeringly high and finally led the World Health Organization to take steps to limit how formula companies could market their products. This is known as the WHO International Code of Marketing of Breast-Milk Substitutes, or the WHO Code for short. The United States as a country did not vote for the WHO Code when it was ratified (the United States was the only country to vote against it) and the United States—unlike some other countries—has not incorporated the WHO Code into the law of the land. But most key U.S. breastfeeding organizations support it.

JUST AS GOOD?

Unfortunately, there are still problems today. Formula has gained a solid place among mothers around the world. Outside the United States, many mothers see formula as the Western way to feed a baby, which they think must make it better than breastfeeding. Unfortunately, women coming to the United States from developing countries often abandon breastfeeding in favor of more "modern" ways of feeding their babies, even if they breastfed their children in their home countries. And many women born in the United States (including many health professionals) are unaware of the health consequences to them and to their babies if they don't breastfeed. So when these women have breastfeeding difficulties, they are more likely to give up.

WILL THE REAL SCIENTIFIC MOTHER PLEASE STAND UP?

In retrospect, we see that the efficacy of science was vastly overestimated. Science did not bring an end to all human suffering. Just when one problem was conquered, another reared its ugly head. For example, when smallpox was virtually eliminated, scientists were then faced with the AIDS epidemic. And even smallpox is reappearing. It

189

was, in many cases, pure hubris to believe that science could create a perfect world.

Losing the human touch. We are also realizing now that we were too quick to abandon many of the old ways that were actually quite effective and indeed probably better than what replaced them. In medicine, there are many examples of this. In recent times, patients have started to protest what seem to them to be a purely mechanistic approach to health and healing. They want to be treated as whole people, not just the sum of body parts. One example of this reaction is the astounding growth of alternative medicine, with herbal medicine being the most visible example. Another example is the burgeoning field of health psychology and the related field of *psychoneuroimmunology*, where researchers have found that people's attitudes, beliefs, and social connections are also vital to survival.

Breastfeeding and survival. Interestingly, science has also come around to the breastfeeding point of view. As we explained in the introduction, thousands of studies have now demonstrated the inferiority of nonhuman milks when compared with breastfeeding. The women who defied the "wisdom" of their day and breastfed their babies were in fact the real scientific mothers, and we are in their debt. These were the mothers who paid attention to their babies' cues, who fed the babies when they were hungry, rocked or carried them when they were cranky, and came to them when they cried. They ignored the experts and listened to their own hearts. On the surface, their approach seems the exact opposite of scientific. But if "scientific" means increasing the likelihood that babies would survive, then they were right on the money.

Cultural Beliefs About Babies and Breastfeeding

Despite the amply demonstrated inferiority of feeding babies nonhuman milks to breastfeeding, scientific mothering is still alive and well. Many of our cultural beliefs that undermine breastfeeding are an outgrowth of both scientific mothering and generations of bottlefeeding. There are many misconceptions that are prominent in our culture about the needs of babies, even though science has soundly disproved them. The next few sections describe some of the beliefs that can be destructive to you and your baby. Know that these have no scientific support, despite the widespread belief to the contrary.

THE IMPORTANCE OF SCHEDULE

As a new mother, you will frequently be asked whether your baby is sleeping through the night and is on some type of regular eating and sleeping schedule. These are purported to be "good" characteristics, while nonregulated eating and sleeping patterns are "bad."

These beliefs about the importance of schedule are based on a couple of erroneous assumptions. First, they assume that all mothers and babies are the same, which they are not (see chapter 6). Second, they fail to take into account babies' legitimate physical needs, such as hunger. As we described in chapter 4, a newborn baby has a stomach the size of a large shooter marble. Your baby is in the best position to tell you whether he is hungry. The use of "ideal feeding schedules" has absolutely no basis in science. That bears saying again: there is no science that supports a feeding schedule for a breastfed baby. When a schedule becomes your principal guide for when to feed your baby, you are no longer reading your baby's feeding cues. The net result is that your baby's instinctive feeding behavior is suppressed. Both you and your baby lose.

THE PARENT MUST BE THE BOSS

This is another belief that we frequently hear from mothers, and it saddens us. This belief often has religious overtones that gravely warn parents to "discipline" their children from the start lest they lose control ("You don't want your child to grow up to be a drug addict, do you?"). This belief depends heavily on some pretty weak logic. We agree that disciplining children is part of the responsibility of parents, no question, but it is absurd to extrapolate from that belief that by feeding your child when he's hungry—especially if he's an infant—you are somehow giving in to your child and making him "willful." A baby who cries when he is hungry is expressing a legitimate physical need, a need that ensures his survival. By crying, a baby is communicating in his most direct and attention-getting way. In terms of how "giving in" to babies sets them up for future behavior problems, science has found the opposite to be true. Babies reared by nonresponsive or harsh parents are significantly more likely to engage in harmful behaviors—including drug abuse. This has been repeatedly demonstrated in dozens of studies. Bottom line: responding to your baby's needs is good for him.

BABIES MANIPULATE ADULTS BY CRYING

This belief is similar to the one described above. It is something, sadly, that we hear from mothers on a regular basis. Mothers often believe that they shouldn't "give in" to their babies because that would be doing what the babies want. Yes, that's precisely it! Remember, crying and fussing are the only ways babies can communicate. Telling you that they want to be fed, changed, or held is a perfectly legitimate behavior. It is not manipulative for your baby to tell you that he needs something that will help him to survive.

Consider this issue another way. Is your baby sophisticated enough to manipulate you? To do this, babies must be able to form what developmental psychologists call a *metacognition*. That is, they must be able to think about what they are thinking ("If I cry, then someone will come"). Babies can't do this until they are many months old. They can't yet conceive of the results of their actions. They just know they need help.

IGNORING A BABY'S CRIES WILL MAKE HIM CRY LESS

As described earlier, this belief maintains that if you want a baby who cries less, you should not respond to his cries, and it is straight out of the philosophy of behaviorism, one of the schools of thought that brought us scientific mothering. Back in its heyday, its practitioners (behaviorists such as John B. Watson in his 1928 book *Psychological Care of the Infant and Child*) told mothers not to hold, touch, or cuddle their babies for fear of spoiling them. Some vestiges of this belief still exist today. In fact, you may be surprised to learn that many students of psychology are still taught this both as undergraduates and graduate students. Again, this is one of those beliefs that doesn't stand up to scientific scrutiny.

In the United States, *longitudinal studies* (studies that follow children's development as they age) have compared mothers who were responsive to their babies during infancy and mothers who were less responsive. The burning question was this: if mothers ignored their babies' cries, would the babies cry less than babies of mothers who responded promptly? Guess what: the responsive mothers had babies who cried less (Bates, Maslin, and Frankel 1985; Crockenberg and McCluskey 1986).

Psychiatrist John Bowlby and developmental psychologist Mary Ainsworth, both founders of *attachment theory*, dedicated their lives to the study of parent-child attachment, the factors that promote it, and what happens when it is not there. In a remarkable paper they wrote together at the end of their careers, they noted that there were two things that promoted secure attachments between parent and child: caregiver proximity and responsivity (Ainsworth and Bowlby 1991). In other words, caregivers (in these studies, usually mothers) needed to be nearby and responsive to their babies' cues.

The importance of responsive parenting has also been demonstrated in cross-cultural research. Research into other cultures is valuable because researchers are often unaware of the values, beliefs, and assumptions that they bring to their research. For example, in the not-too-distant past, it was difficult to study breastfeeding mothers in this culture because they were such a small minority of women. Many of the standards we used to measure normal infant development (such as growth charts) were based on babies who were formula fed. That is changing, but it goes to show how pervasive the influence of culture is. When researchers went into completely different cultures, many of the things the researchers believed were normal were quickly exposed as being part of their culture, not universal human traits. You might be surprised to learn that not all human babies regularly cry. That's what research on a tribe called the !Kung found.

The !Kung are a traditional culture and tribe who are considered to be hunter-gatherers. For many, it has been instructive to observe their childrearing strategies. In this culture, babies sleep with their mothers. They are held most of the time because there is no safe place to set them down. Mothers often "wear" babies by placing them in a carrier on their bodies, where the babies have near constant access to their mothers' breasts and breastfeed at will. And they rarely cry. As toddlers, these babies are more independent than their counterparts in the United States (Konner 1976).

This is just one of many examples in the literature. When studying other cultures, we don't want to assume that they do everything better than we do, but neither do we want to reject what they do as being too "primitive." Other cultures can be instructive—especially when they haven't been touched by industrialization and scientific mothering. So many tenets of scientific mothering have been refuted that any advice based on its beliefs bears close scrutiny.

General Ignorance of Breastfeeding

Unfortunately, scientific mothering is not the only cultural force that can interfere with breastfeeding. Ignorance is another influential force undermining the natural laws of breastfeeding. An obvious consequence of this ignorance, combined with poor breastfeeding management, is the sharp drop-off of exclusive breastfeeding after birth. According to the U.S. Centers for Disease Control and Prevention, in 2006, 50 percent of U.S. mothers were exclusively breastfeeding at one week, but by four months, that number dropped to 26 percent (CDC 2010).

Ignorance about breastfeeding has its roots in our familiarity with bottlefeeding. As we have explained, breastfeeding is best learned by watching others do it as a normal part of daily life. But those of us who grew up exposed primarily to bottlefeeding have bottlefeeding norms ingrained in our thinking, consciously or unconsciously, and these bottlefeeding expectations may need to be unlearned.

APPLYING BOTTLEFEEDING NORMS

Many women approach breastfeeding thinking, either consciously or subconsciously, that they can use what they know about bottlefeeding to breastfeed. Unfortunately, there are enough basic differences that this does not usually work well.

Using bottlefeeding technique to breastfeed. As an example, in the early 1980s, many mothers were instructed to hold their babies in their arms for breastfeeding with their babies facing the ceiling (a bottlefeeding position). They were then told to tickle the baby's cheek with their nipple until baby turned his head toward the breast, and then to let the baby latch on. To understand how difficult it is to feed in this position, try turning your head all the way to one side and swallowing. Using a bottlefeeding position to breastfeed made it difficult for babies. This position also made breastfeeding difficult for mothers because when babies fed with their heads turned, they pulled on the nipple, causing pain and trauma. This was no doubt one factor contributing to the common misconception that nipple trauma is normal for breastfeeding mothers (not so!).

As we'll explain more fully in the section "They Go with What They Know" (toward the end of this chapter), health care providers often have poor or outdated information about breastfeeding. Medical or nursing school training still offers very little instruction in breastfeeding, so health care providers often must fall back on their own experiences—good or bad—when advising mothers about breastfeeding. This means that the people new mothers tend to turn to first, doctors and nurses, usually know little about how to manage common breastfeeding challenges. We wish we had a nickel for every new mother with nipple trauma who started their conversation with, "The nurses in the hospital told me my latch is fine." In most cases, adjusting the "fine" latch proved to be the key to eliminating the nipple pain.

Normal feeding patterns. We described in chapters 4 and 5 the normal breastfeeding patterns of healthy newborns. But for those of us more familiar with bottlefeeding, breastfeeding norms may not feel normal at all. As we explained, babies fed by bottle (no matter what is in the bottle) tend to take more at a feeding and feed fewer times per day: bottlefed newborns tend to feed six to eight times per day, whereas breastfeeding newborns tend to feed more like eight to twelve times per day. Because of the dynamics of the delivery system, bottlefeeding establishes an overfeeding pattern early in life. While not necessarily healthy, bottlefeeding norms may still feel normal if that's what you're used to. As we said earlier, new parents are still encouraged by many to use feeding schedules. Although this can work for bottlefed babies, scheduling can sometimes lead to breastfeeding problems such as milk-production issues and slow weight gain, which we discussed in detail in chapter 6.

Rigid feeding schedules can also lead to other breastfeeding problems. We know a lactation consultant who made a home visit to a mother just discharged from the hospital whose baby was not latching on. When the consultant arrived, the baby was sound asleep. While the consultant was filling out the paperwork, the baby started to stir. The consultant said, "Why don't we come back to the paperwork later and work with the baby now. He acts as if he's ready to feed." The mother looked at the clock and said, "No. It's not time to breastfeed yet." The mother explained that she had been told at the hospital to breastfeed every three hours. She took these instructions literally and had been ignoring her baby's cues and cries, picking him up and trying to breastfeed on the dot of the third hour. At every "feeding time" the baby was either sound asleep or screaming so hard that the mother couldn't calm him to feed. The solution to her problem was very simple. As soon as she began breastfeeding whenever her baby showed early feeding cues (rooting, hand to mouth), breastfeeding went smoothly.

Few mothers approach breastfeeding as literally and rigidly as this mother, but her story is instructive. Bottlefeeding by the clock can work because a reluctant feeder can sometimes be "forced" to feed by pushing the firm bottle nipple into the back of baby's mouth, which triggers active sucking. But a baby who is not ready to breastfeed cannot be forced to. The baby must be willing and ready to draw the soft breast back to the comfort zone. Like a dance, breastfeeding only works if both people cooperate. Breastfeeding may be nature's first lesson in healthy human interactions.

Commercial Pressures

Another cultural force that undermines breastfeeding is commercial pressure. Formula manufacturing is a multibillion-dollar industry. As for any business, a primary goal of formula companies is to keep and increase market share. Unfortunately, as the formula industry's market share rises, breastfeeding decreases and the health of mothers and babies suffers.

FORMULA MARKETING AIMED AT PARENTS

Amazing as it may seem to those of us in the United States, prior to 1991 there were no magazine ads or television commercials for infant formula in this country. Print ads were the only advertising for formula, and they appeared only in medical journals that were directed at doctors. However, once formula advertising started to be directed at parents, a whole new challenge to breastfeeding came into being. Mothers may run into this advertising in surprising places. For example, in a recent article on breastfeeding on WebMD, there was an embedded slide show called "Breastfeeding Hints and Hurdles." There was some accurate information in it. But there was also a lot of misinformation that could cause breastfeeding to fail (WebMD 2010). This slide show was funded by Gerber and offered mothers coupons and other incentives for buying formula. (A full description of this slide show is on our website at www. breastfeedingmadesimple; see "Deconstructing Gerber.")

Earlier in this chapter, we mentioned the WHO Code, which was created to stop the marketing of infant formula to the general public. The WHO Code was needed because of the many deaths resulting from unethical formula marketing practices in developing nations. But the WHO Code was not meant only for developing nations. From a public-health perspective, it makes sense to eliminate direct marketing of formula to consumers everywhere.

Although the United States was the only country to vote against the WHO Code, for many years the formula companies abided by it by not advertising directly to parents. However, in 1991, Gerber opened the floodgates with its direct marketing campaign to consumers. Now all major formula manufacturers devote some of their considerable marketing budgets to print and television ads for parents. In the United States, pregnant women are bombarded with these formula ads, and it is the rare family that does not receive coupons by mail for discounts on infant formula, cases of formula delivered directly to their door, and formula marketing bags given "free" at hospitals when they give birth. (Hospitals—supposedly promoters of public health—are rewarded financially for their role as formula endorsers and marketers.)

Are formula marketing bags really "free"? These bags are actually far from "free," even to families who exclusively formula feed. They contain the most expensive infant formulas, because market research has found that once a formula is given, 95 percent of parents are unlikely to switch to another for fear their baby might have a reaction to it (http://banthebags.org/bb-pdf/onepage.pdf). The price difference between this expensive formula and the generic store brands over a baby's first year is about US$700, the real cost to families of this "free" bag.

We are happy to report, however, that the practice of giving formula marketing bags to new parents may be changing. Currently, in New York City, for example, public hospitals are not allowed to provide free formula to new parents. Moreover, the U.S. WIC government food-subsidy program for low-income families now offers as an incentive a premium food package to mothers who exclusively breastfeed.

Most people firmly believe (despite much research to the contrary) that they are not influenced by marketing. But there is no doubt that commercial pressures have done much to normalize the use of infant formula and thereby undermine breastfeeding. In the United States today, it is the rare baby who does not receive at least some infant formula.

TAPPING INTO NEW-PARENT ANXIETY

The following is just one example of how vulnerable new parents are targeted by formula companies to the detriment of breastfeeding.

In 2003 at a conference for lactation professionals, Virginia Tech English professor Bernice Hausman provided a fascinating analysis of formula marketing strategies (Hausman 2003). During her fifth month of pregnancy, Hausman began receiving formula marketing materials. In the mailing that arrived just before her baby was due, she received formula coupons and a chart with the following headings:

My baby has...	Which could mean...	Type of formula
Problems with gas	Baby reacts to lactose	Enfamil Lactose-Free

Along with "Problems with gas," other conditions in the "My baby has..." column included "Restless sleep," "Fussy times," and even "Absence of a regular schedule." The second column interpreted the baby's behavior, and the third column listed which of the "Enfamil Family of Formulas" provided a solution to the baby's "problem." Of course, human milk or breastfeeding were mentioned nowhere on the chart.

This approach feeds into new parents' normal insecurities in order to sell formula. Absence of a regular schedule, fussy periods, restless sleep, and gas are all normal aspects of infancy. If formula companies successfully convince new parents that these are problems in need of a solution, they are halfway down the slippery slope to solving their problem with "the right formula." (Of course, if someone were paid to market breastfeeding using this strategy, a similar chart would include problems we know to be related to formula use, such as constipation, allergy, illness, and digestive problems, with breastfeeding listed as the solution for them all.)

These formula-marketing materials also feed into the expectations created by scientific mothering, such as new parents' desire for their babies to sleep well, feed at predictable intervals, and never act fussy. They also feed into the cultural expectation many new parents have that in order to meet their baby's needs, they must buy a wide variety of consumer products. As Hausman noted: "Problems are addressed through the purchase of goods.... Thus one goal of formula promotion materials is to identify baby behavior as problems that can be solved through a specific, informed purchase" (Hausman 2003).

Breastfeeding and the Medical Community

Although some progress has been made in recent years, some of the greatest obstacles to normal breastfeeding after birth come from what appears on the face of it to be an unlikely source: the medical community. These obstacles are due in part to the inertia of institutions ("We've always done it this way") after generations of formula feeding, but commercial pressures also play a role here.

A BOTTLEFEEDING MENTALITY

Like many in the United States, medical professionals today, by and large, tend to have a "bottlefeeding mentality" because of their greater familiarity with formula feeding. The U.S. medical community is so well educated about formula and so poorly educated about breastfeeding that they often unknowingly undermine the latter.

THEY GO WITH WHAT THEY KNOW

Despite their sincere desire to help, medical providers tend to go with the familiar. The formula industry makes sure that doctors and nurses learn about formula feeding both during medical school and after. As part of their marketing efforts, the industry sponsors meals with free educational seminars and even perks such as cruises. But this is changing. Many hospitals and medical schools have recently implemented policies banning the influence of for-profit companies in medical education. Initially, many of these efforts were an attempt to curb the influence of pharmaceutical manufacturers. But these policies also cover the marketing of formula. And many formula companies are subsidiaries of pharmaceutical companies.

Unfortunately, there is still much to do. Doctors we know have also received unlimited supplies of free formula for their own babies because formula company representatives know that these doctors can be very influential in encouraging their patients to use formula.

Because they are well-trained in bottlefeeding, when doctors and nurses are unsure about how to help a new mother make breastfeeding work, they often suggest switching to or supplementing with formula rather than referring a mother to a specialist for breastfeeding help, as they would with most other health issues. Many health professionals fed their own children formula, which can make it more difficult for them to accept the importance of breastfeeding.

Those doctors and nurses who do know about breastfeeding only learn about it if they happen to have a special interest in it. Then they must pursue their learning on their own and at their own expense. Another way some health care providers learn about breastfeeding is if they or their spouse breastfeed. A major overhaul is desperately needed in breastfeeding education for doctors and nurses.

THE OVERUSE OF FORMULA

An outgrowth of this bottlefeeding mentality is the gross overuse of formula. Please don't misunderstand us here. Formula can a blessing in the rare cases in which it is truly needed. This need is the greatest in the United States and in parts of the world where donor human milk is only available on a limited basis for babies with serious health problems. In some parts of the world, like Scandinavia and Brazil, many babies whose mothers' milk is unavailable are routinely fed donor human milk from milk banks, avoiding the negative health outcomes of nonhuman milks.

FORMULA ADVOCATES

If you have not yet given birth and you prefer your baby not be given formula, be prepared. Depending upon the institution, formula supplementation may not only be routine, it may also be very difficult to prevent. As one lactation consultant writes:

> In a survey I conducted in Utah, 25 percent of the nurses felt formula was so important to a baby's well-being that they would give formula even if the physician or mother specifically said not to.
>
> By experience I learned that there are some staff members who feel so sorry for the breastfed babies (who seem to get fed so little compared to formula-fed babies) that they will take any opportunity to feed them, truly feeling that they are looking out for the babies' welfare better than the misguided mothers and doctors who want the baby to be exclusively breastfed. They can be strengthened in this belief if there is one physician who vocalizes the same beliefs, though he be only one physician of many (Helm, 2004).

As we described in the introduction, the premature introduction of nonhuman milks can put your baby at risk for allergies and a variety of other health problems. Despite its overuse, formula is not benign to either breastfeeding or to your baby. It may sometimes be necessary, but most often it is given unnecessarily. In some birthing facilities, nurses know so little about normal breastfeeding that they believe newborns' desire to feed long and often in the early days means that these babies need formula supplements. Many new mothers are undermined in their desire to exclusively breastfeed by health care providers who tell them they don't have enough milk.

HOW TO AVOID FORMULA EXPOSURE

If you give birth in a hospital and want to avoid exposing your baby to formula, the best way is to take advantage of the rooming-in option and keep your baby with you at all times. If that isn't possible, the next best thing is to get an order of "no supplements" in writing from your baby's health care provider. If your baby's usual health care provider is not on staff where you will be giving birth, your baby will be assigned a doctor on staff and that doctor's orders will be followed until your baby is discharged. In this case, you'll need to get a no-supplement order in writing from the doctor on staff. It isn't enough for the doctor to promise this verbally. If your baby's doctor's orders include routine supplementation, you need to go to the hospital with your exception in writing, signed by the doctor, and give copies to those caring for your baby. If you don't, your baby may be given supplements until the doctor says otherwise.

Summary

As you can see, there are some major forces at work that can undermine breastfeeding. At one point in the not-too-distant past, breastfeeding was in danger of dying out in the United States. Breastfeeding had no backing from major scientific organizations (that has certainly changed!) and had no international organizations working for its success. The only thing it did have was the very real health drawbacks of other methods of infant feeding.

Yet despite all the forces that have conspired against breastfeeding, breastfeeding rates are continuing to rise in the United States, increasing an average of about 1 percent annually over the past decade (CDC

2010). Knowing about the forces that interfere with the laws of breast-feeding is important in neutralizing their influence. After all, knowledge is power. Understanding these dynamics can help you distinguish good advice from bad advice and the good breastfeeding information from the questionable. This knowledge gives you a better perspective from which to make important decisions for you, your baby, and your whole family.

PART II

Applying the Laws

CHAPTER 9

Daily Life with Your Breastfeeding Baby

Having a baby changes every aspect of your life. But you probably already know that! You may sometimes long for your former life B.C.—before children. Your B.C. days may be over, but you can embrace a new normal that includes life with your baby. As a breastfeeding woman, you can still be a part of the wider world. This chapter will help you to make this transition.

Reentering the World with Your Breastfeeding Baby

Reentering the world means being out and about with your baby. Breastfeeding can simplify this. There may also be times when you need to be away from your baby. We offer some suggestions on how you can do both.

As a new mother, you may wonder about how best to handle feedings when you and your baby venture out of the house. No one thinks twice about giving a baby a bottle in public. Yet many women worry about offending others by breastfeeding. What are some of your options when breastfeeding away from home?

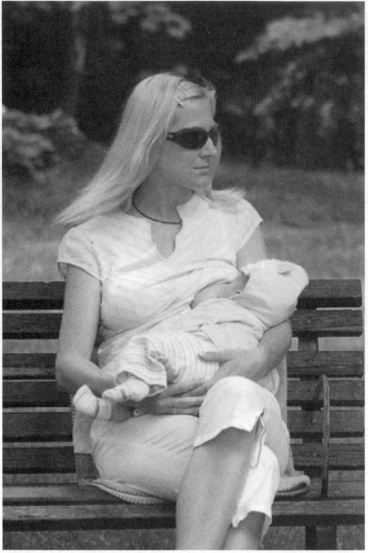

With practice, you can feel comfortable breastfeeding anywhere.

You Can Breastfeed Anywhere

If you feel nervous about breastfeeding in public, learning how to feed your baby discreetly can help. Some mothers drape a blanket over one shoulder to cover the baby. Others wrap the baby in the blanket and pull the corner up over their breast. This allows you to see your baby, and it doesn't cover the baby's head and face, which bothers some babies. There are also commercially sold nursing coverups.

Discreet breastfeeding is easier if you wear a two-piece outfit. You can lift your top from the bottom, with your baby's body covering any exposed skin. Jackets, cardigan sweaters, and overblouses also provide extra coverage. There are also special breastfeeding fashions with openings and panels to make discreet nursing even easier. (See our website at www.breastfeedingmadesimple.com for additional information.) Many women have gained confidence by practicing in front of a mirror or having a partner take a look.

Baby slings can also be helpful. Although at this writing, one brand of sling has been recalled due to safety concerns, there are many safe brands on the market. Many mothers find nursing a baby in a sling the height of ease and modesty because they either use the tail of the sling as a cover-up or pull up the extra fabric of the sling to cover the baby. This allows them to breastfeed while walking around public places with no one the wiser.

You Can Find a Private Place

Even mothers who are usually comfortable breastfeeding in public may sometimes prefer more privacy. Some shopping centers and other public areas offer special areas for breastfeeding moms. Other options include changing rooms, lounges, or benches in a quiet part of the mall. To make breastfeeding less obvious in a restaurant, you may choose to sit at a table in the back of the restaurant, with your back toward the front. A restroom is probably the least desirable place to breastfeed (it's not a great place for anyone to eat, especially a baby). But it can be an option, if needed.

Family gatherings may also present a challenge, especially if you're the first one in your family to breastfeed. Depending on those in attendance, you may choose to breastfeed in another room—or not. Some mothers will abide by others' preferences in someone else's home, but not when in their own homes. With more exposure (no pun intended!), many families gain a greater comfort level with breastfeeding.

Many U.S. States Have Breastfeeding Laws

A number of U.S. states have passed laws protecting a woman's right to breastfeed in public. These laws came about because some women were harassed for breastfeeding in restaurants, shopping malls, and even doctors' offices. These laws do not require discreet breastfeeding, as they rightly assume that there's nothing indecent about feeding your baby. (It's the normal way for a baby to eat!) And consider the recent campaign on Facebook: "Hey, Facebook. Breastfeeding is not obscene." This campaign was launched after pictures of breastfeeding mothers were banned from Facebook. After protest from Facebook users, that ban has been lifted.

Laws protecting breastfeeding in public were necessary because sometimes even discreetly breastfeeding mothers were hassled, asked to leave restaurants, and even escorted off of airplanes when someone discovered that they were breastfeeding. To see if your state has such a law, refer to our website (www.breastfeedingmadesimple.com) for a listing.

Away from Your Baby

In chapter 2, we explained why a mother's body is a baby's natural habitat and that separation is physically stressful for babies. In chapter 5, we described different types of mammalian feeding patterns and concluded that humans are carry mammals, requiring constant carrying and feeding. Understanding human biology gives you a great perspective on your baby. It helps you appreciate why she gets so upset when you put her down and why skin-to-skin contact with you gives her such pleasure.

Sorting Out Your Feelings

But understanding it and living it may be an entirely different matter. Perhaps you have decided to do whatever it takes to never miss a breastfeeding. Maybe you wish you could live your life that way, but practicalities interfere. It could be that you consider exclusive breastfeeding interesting to think about but have no desire to be with your baby 24/7. Whatever your situation or your preference, you can still make breastfeeding work.

How to Handle Times Apart

There are a number of ways to handle breastfeeding during the times you and your baby are apart:

- *Time your outings so that you don't miss feedings.* If your baby is somewhat regular in her breastfeeding patterns, you may be able to slip out between feedings without having to leave any milk behind.

- *Make arrangements to have your baby brought to you at feeding times.* Try to be creative when thinking of ways to get your baby to you for feeding. You may have more latitude than you think. While not every setting is appropriate for a baby, it may be possible to have someone bring the baby to you when it's time to breastfeed.

- *Follow your heart.* This is ultimately your decision. If you do not want to be away from your baby, don't let others pressure you to. There's nothing that says being away is necessary for everyone. And if you need or want to be away, that's your decision, too.

- *This too shall pass.* It's so easy to lose perspective during the intense early months when you're adjusting to motherhood. Some women worry that this stage of intense mothering will last forever. As two experienced mothers, we can tell you that this stage actually goes by pretty quickly. But it doesn't necessarily feel that way at the time. When you allow yourself to relish to the fullest the closeness and intimacy you can have with your baby, you gain a depth and a richness in your life that wasn't there before you had children. Think of this intense time as an opportunity for personal growth. Instead of trying to hurry this phase along or believing the cultural messages that you "need" to get away from your baby, try as much as possible to relax and enjoy this time together.

- *In almost every situation, it's still possible to breastfeed.* Even mothers who need to be away from their babies for extended periods (such as women who work full-time and travel or are active-duty military) can still maintain their milk production when they are away and breastfeed when they are with their babies.

- *Leave your milk for your baby.* If you will be away at a feeding time, you can leave some expressed milk for your baby. If you're gone longer than your baby's longest sleep stretch or your breasts start to feel full, you'll also need to express your milk while you are gone to keep up your milk production and to prevent mastitis.

- *Leave formula for your baby.* If you prefer not to leave your milk, or for some reason cannot, there is always the option of giving formula while you're away. As we've said throughout, some breastfeeding is always better than none.

If You Plan to Use Bottles

If your baby is older than one month of age and you need to be away, chances are that your caregiver will feed your baby with a bottle (see chapter 11 for alternatives for babies younger than one month of age). Bottles are the most common alternative to the breast in developed countries. Bottles are familiar. They are readily available and inexpensive. But bottles are not without controversy. One concern is that babies may come to prefer bottles and then have difficulty going back to the breast, especially if bottles are given during the first month. Some people call this *nipple confusion.* For some babies, this can be a legitimate concern. However, most babies go to the breast just fine even when they've had bottles. Unfortunately, babies are not born with labels to tell you which ones are easily confused and which ones are not. If you're planning to use bottles, here are some strategies that are less likely to compromise breastfeeding:

- *Wait until your baby's about three to four weeks old.* Despite what many people say, studies show it doesn't really seem to matter how late you start bottlefeeding. Approximately 70 percent of babies take a bottle easily whether you start at one month, two months, or even three to six months. Another 26 percent of babies require some patience and persistence to accept a bottle. And a few babies (about 4 percent) refuse a bottle no matter what (Kearney and Cronenwett 1991). But keep in mind that babies can also be fed with a cup, spoon, or dropper (see chapter 11).

- *Have someone else give the bottle.* Your baby may not be willing to take a bottle from you because she's smart enough to know she could be nursing instead. She may not take a bottle if you are even in the building. Have the caregiver try giving a bottle for the first time when baby is not too hungry. If the baby won't take the bottle in the nursing position, try other positions. A good long-term strategy for a baby who will be receiving regular bottles is to confine bottlefeeding to the caregiver, having mom do only breastfeeding.

- *Pick a bottle your baby likes with as slow-flow a nipple as possible.* The best bottle is the type your baby likes. Start by buying several types of bottles and nipples and see how your baby responds to them. Babies have mouths of different shapes and sizes, so don't buy too many of one kind of bottle and nipple until you're sure your baby is okay with it. The reason a slow-flow nipple is a better choice for a breastfeeding baby (no matter what her age) is that like adults, the slower a baby feeds, the sooner she will feel full. Being able to satisfy the baby with a smaller amount of expressed milk decreases the amount you have to express and store for a feeding when you and your baby are apart. Each bottle manufacturer has a different definition of "slow flow," so it may be best to buy several brands, fill the bottles with water, and turn them upside down. You'll be amazed at how different the flow rates are. Choose the slowest flow that your baby will accept.

Employment Outside the Home

The question of whether to work outside the home is one that many mothers wrestle with. Fortunately, you can continue breastfeeding even if you and your baby are regularly apart. In this case, to meet your breastfeeding goals, it helps to plan ahead.

BEFORE GOING BACK TO WORK

Advance planning before you head back to work can help smooth this transition. Decide on your breastfeeding goals. Breastfeeding doesn't have to be all or nothing. Your choices include the following:

- maintaining full milk production and supplying only mother's milk for the feedings you and your baby are apart

- supplying as much mother's milk as is convenient, using formula as needed

- supplementing with formula while away; breastfeeding when together

Consider your work options. The number of hours you work and the type of work you do can affect breastfeeding. Will you work full-time or part-time? How old will baby be when you return to work? Waiting until your baby is at least three months old can improve your chances of keeping up your milk production long term. Can you work from home? Are there job-sharing options? Is there flextime? Can you take your baby to work? Can baby be brought to you at work for feedings? See our website (www.breastfeedingmadesimple.com) for more employment options.

Find a breastfeeding-friendly caregiver. Look for a caregiver supportive of breastfeeding. Finding one close to work (rather than close to home) might allow you to breastfeed baby at breaks by either going to your baby or having your baby brought to you. If you breastfeed at the caregiver's before leaving for work and immediately when you arrive to pick up your baby, it also cuts down on your time apart, decreasing the amount of milk needed while you're away.

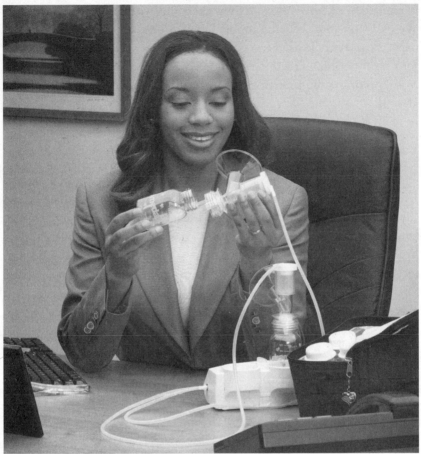

The Ameda Purely Yours breast pump is a good choice for women employed full-time who plan to pump at work. (©2010 Ameda Breastfeeding Products, used with permission of Ameda, Lincolnshire, IL)

Build your supply of expressed milk. Allow at least three to four weeks before starting back to work to get practiced with your method of milk expression and to start storing milk. Keep in mind that once at work, the milk you express one day can be left for the next day. If you express milk just once a day for three weeks, you'll have enough milk for your first day back to work and a good reserve.

215

Make note of how many times each day your baby breastfeeds.
We call this your "magic number." It is a clue to your breast storage
capacity and can be used as a guide for how many times in each twenty-
four-hour period you will need to drain your breasts (by breastfeeding
or expressing milk) to maintain your milk production once you're back
at work.

MAKE ARRANGEMENTS AT WORK

Before you return to work, talk with your employer about what you
will need in order to continue to breastfeed. Let your company know
that your continuing to breastfeed benefits them. When companies
support breastfeeding, women return to work more quickly, use fewer
health care dollars, take fewer sick days, and report greater job satisfaction, resulting in reduced staff turnover. (See the following website
for full-color brochures created by the U.S. government that you can
share with your employer: "The Business Case for Breastfeeding" at
www.womenshealth.gov/breastfeeding/programs/business-case/.) Here
is some of what you will need to arrange at your workplace:

- *Find a place to express.* You will need a place to express your
  milk where you can relax and have some privacy. Ask if you
  can use a private office, conference room, storage room, or
  lounge. A bathroom is not ideal because it isn't sanitary. But
  if it's your only option, you can make it work. If you're using
  a breast pump and an electrical outlet is not available, some
  quality breast pumps can be powered by batteries, battery
  packs, or even car adapters.

- *Allow twenty minutes per session.* If you are using a double
  pump, allow ten to fifteen minutes per pumping session and
  five minutes for clean-up. If you plan to keep up full milk
  production and provide your baby exclusively with your
  milk, divide the number of hours away from baby, including
  travel time, by three (for example, nine hours away means
  three pumpings). Depending on their breast storage capacity (see chapter 6), some mothers can provide enough milk
  with fewer pumping sessions.

216

- *Decide on a place to store milk.* You can store your milk at room temperature for up to four to six hours. However, if you are away for longer than this, you'll need to cool your milk. Cooling choices include a separate cooler compartment in your pump case, a separate cooler bag, or a refrigerator. Fresh and cooled batches of milk can be combined (though fresh milk must be cooled before being added to frozen milk). Human milk is not a biohazard, and no unusual precautions are needed.

CHOOSING A METHOD OF EXPRESSION

If you are planning to supply your milk while you're away, another decision you'll need to make is how to express your milk. For more information, see "Expressing and Storing Milk," later in this chapter.

If you choose to use a breast pump, see the following suggestions for pumps best suited for full- and part-time work. The type of pump most likely to meet your needs will depend upon the amount of time you're away from your baby.

Away from baby full-time. If your goal is to keep up your milk production and you'll be away from baby for feedings thirty to forty-plus hours per week, your choices include Ameda or Medela rental pumps. Or you may purchase the Ameda Purely Yours models or one of the Medela Pump In Styles. These pumps provide you with stimulation similar to a baby actively nursing (forty to sixty suction-and-release cycles per minute). Most women find that using a pump that is limited to fewer cycles leads to a gradually decreasing milk production. When pricing pumps, keep in mind that formula costs between US$100–$250 per month. A good pump is an investment that pays back many times over.

Away from baby part-time. If you'll be working part-time, you'll miss fewer feedings and have more options in terms of pumps. The pumps described above will work well, but if you plan to pump less than once a day, consider pumps that provide fewer cycles per minute. If your number of work hours is very limited, you may even do well with a good manual pump.

ONCE YOU'RE BACK AT WORK

To keep up your milk production over the long term, don't forget Law 6: *More milk out equals more milk made.*

Keep an eye on how many times every twenty-four hours you drain your breasts. Remember your "magic number"? This is the average number of times your baby breastfeeds every twenty-four hours while you are at home. To keep your milk production steady over the long term, try to match it with your total number of breastfeedings plus pumpings per day. As we explained in chapter 6, your breast storage capacity determines, in part, how long you can go between feedings before your breasts become full, which slows your milk production. Because breast storage capacity varies among mothers, so does the "magic number."

Plan to provide most of your baby's milk directly from the breast. When we talk to mothers who have returned to work and are struggling with milk production, we've found that many of them are pumping as often as recommended at work but not breastfeeding enough when they're with their babies. Their "magic number" (number of breast drainings per day) decreases along with their milk production. Mothers who were breastfeeding eight times per day before they returned to work may be pumping three times at their worksite but only breastfeeding twice or three times each day. This may be because the baby is sleeping more at night or due to issues with their daily routine (see the next section). In other words, during times when they could be breastfeeding, they're not. In practical terms, this means that the baby needs more expressed milk while mother and baby are apart, which mothers have to work harder to provide. When back at work, keep in mind that your baby will continue to need a fixed amount of about 30 oz. (900 ml) on average per day. The more of those ounces your baby gets directly from the breast while you're together, the less milk you need to express. The opposite is true, too. The less milk the baby gets from the breast, the more milk she'll need while you're at work.

Plan your daily routine as if milk production matters. For this reason, a good goal is to breastfeed your baby as much as possible when you're together to reduce the amount of expressed milk needed. Consider breastfeeding twice in the morning: once when you wake up, and again right before you leave her. Breastfeed as soon as you see your baby after work. If she seems hungry right before you arrive, suggest the caregiver give as little milk as possible until you get there. If your baby starts sleeping longer at night and the overall number of breast drainings decreases, think about when you can fit in more breastfeedings at other times. If your baby sleeps for long stretches at night, wake her to breastfeed (or get up at night to express your milk).

One mother we talked to was frustrated because her baby was taking 20 oz. (600 ml) of expressed milk during her eight-hour work day and she couldn't keep up. (Her baby was taking twice as much milk as expected: two-thirds of her daily milk intake of 30 oz. [900 ml] during one-third of her twenty-four-hour day.) When we asked about her daily routine, she explained that her baby was fed a 5 oz. (150 ml) bottle of expressed milk as soon as she arrived at daycare, two more 5 oz. bottles (10 oz., or 300 ml) bottles during the day, and one more right before she picked her up so that she wouldn't be hungry on the trip home. Needless to say, that baby wasn't very interested in breastfeeding when they got home. All this mother needed to do to cut nearly in half the amount of expressed milk she needed while at work was to breastfeed before leaving her baby at daycare and to ask the caregiver to feed only a little milk before the mother got there to breastfeed. That small adjustment in daily routine decreased her baby's need for expressed milk by about 10 oz. (300 ml).

Know how much milk your baby needs. When mother and baby are apart for eight to twelve hours per day, most one- to six-month-old babies will need, on average, 10–15 oz. (300–450 ml) of milk. (Those numbers come from dividing the 30 oz. [900 ml] your baby needs daily by one-third for eight hours and one-half for twelve hours.) If a baby is taking much more than this, it may be because she is making up for less mother's milk at home. Or maybe there is too much milk in the bottle, and milk is being discarded after feedings. Maybe the caregiver is overfeeding the baby to decrease the time she spends holding and interacting with her. There is usually a reason, and often adjustments can be made that can decrease the amount of milk needed and make your life easier.

Learn how to encourage milk flow when pumping. In addition to focusing on the milk the baby takes, it may also help to maximize the milk you express. Work can sometimes be stressful, and stress can inhibit milk release, slowing milk flow. If you sit down to pump and the milk is not flowing, see "Expressing to Store Milk" (later in this chapter) for tips.

Know how to stop leaks. Not all women leak. If you do, use nursing pads or LilyPadz, a silicone product that applies gentle pressure to your nipples to stop milk flow (see our Resources section). You can also wear patterned blouses instead of solids, to camouflage, or have a cardigan sweater or jacket handy as a cover up. Regular milk expression will minimize leaking, but if you feel a leak starting, you can stop the flow by discreetly applying pressure to the nipples with your forearms.

Know when and how to increase your milk production. If your milk production slows, you should be able to increase it, especially if you act on it right away. Don't wait. Read "Low Milk Production" in chapter 10 on ways to increase your milk production.

Lifestyle Issues

Breastfeeding evolved as a normal part of life. That means there isn't a long list of rules you must follow to make it work, just the basic principles we described in part 1. The following additional information relates to commonly asked questions about lifestyle issues.

Food, Drink, and Other Consumables

Contrary to popular belief, there are no foods that you should eat or avoid while you're breastfeeding. You don't have to drink milk, for example, to make milk.

EVERYTHING IN MODERATION

Your body has the amazing ability to make milk out of anything you eat—pizza, roast beef, or garbanzo beans. Similarly, there are no specific foods all nursing mothers must avoid. Most mothers can eat chocolate, spicy foods, onions, garlic, broccoli, cabbage. The key is—everything in moderation. Many countries (for instance, Thailand and Mexico) have spicy and flavorful cuisines. Mothers in these countries eat spicy foods while breastfeeding with no ill effects on their babies. Enjoy!

Eat to hunger. Extra calories do not seem to be as important as was once believed. Just eat to hunger. The fat stores you acquired during pregnancy provide much of the fuel needed to establish milk production. Research also indicates that your metabolism may be more efficient while nursing than at other times, reducing your need for extra calories (Illingsworth et al. 1986; Hammond 1997). If you are more active, you will need more calories—but you will also feel hungrier.

You can diet while breastfeeding. In fact, this may be a very good time (formula-feeding mothers tend to lose weight more slowly than those who breastfeed). **Note:** It's best to go slowly and lose weight gradually. Any diet plan should include at least 1,800 calories a day.

If your baby seems to be reacting to something in your diet. Sometimes mothers wonder whether something they've eaten is affecting their babies. If you are concerned, keep in mind that almost all babies have fussy periods. Your baby's fussiness is probably unrelated to your diet, especially if you don't also see other physical signs of allergy or sensitivity, such as a rash, congestion, or digestive upset. If you suspect a food is affecting her, try eliminating that food from your diet. It may take a couple of weeks for you to notice a difference. For example, cow's milk and dairy, the most common cause of problems, takes two weeks or so to clear. After you've eliminated a food, try reintroducing it. The most likely culprits in causing allergy are protein foods such as dairy, soy, egg white, peanuts, meat, and fish. Only diet elimination trials will tell you for sure.

Drink to thirst. How much fluid should you drink while breastfeeding? *Drink to thirst* is the simple guideline. Despite the common belief to the contrary, research has not yet found a connection between a mother's fluid intake and her milk production. If your urine is dark yellow, you need more fluids. To make it easy to get a drink when thirsty, keep a container of water or juice at your usual nursing spot.

CAFFEINE, ALCOHOL, AND CIGARETTES

When it comes to caffeine, alcohol, and cigarettes, again, moderation is important.

Caffeine. You may have abstained from caffeine during pregnancy, but there's no need to do so while breastfeeding. Research indicates that a mother can consume up to five cups of coffee before her breastfeeding baby is affected (Nehlig and Debry 1994). One or two cups of coffee or other caffeinated drinks per day will not cause a problem for most breastfeeding mothers and babies.

Alcohol. An occasional beer or glass of wine is also acceptable while breastfeeding. Moderate to heavy drinking would put a baby at risk. But occasional exposure to alcohol through the milk has not been found to be harmful. If you feel strongly that you don't want your baby exposed to any alcohol, you can simply allow time for it to clear from your system. For example, the alcohol from one glass of beer or wine is out of the milk of a 120 lb. woman within two to three hours (Schulte 1995). You don't need to express your milk for the alcohol to pass out of it—alcohol leaves your milk automatically as blood alcohol levels decrease. If a breastfeeding mother has a stronger drink or more than one glass of beer or wine, it would take much longer for her milk to be free of alcohol.

Smoking. Even if you smoke, it is still better for you to breastfeed your baby than not. The benefits of human milk far outweigh any risk associated with nicotine exposure. But there are risks associated with exposing your baby to second-hand smoke. **Note:** Don't smoke around your baby or let others do so, as this can increase the risk of SIDS. And try to cut down on the number of cigarettes you smoke in a day. The fewer cigarettes you smoke, the better it is for you and your baby.

Exercise and Personal Grooming

There are many benefits to exercising after you have a baby. It reduces stress and depression, makes you feel better, and aids in weight loss. Similarly, being able to engage in grooming routines will help you feel better and bring a renewed sense of normalcy to your life.

YOU CAN EXERCISE

Sometimes mothers wonder whether it's okay to exercise while breastfeeding. The short answer is yes. One early study raised a concern about whether enough of a substance called lactic acid accumulated in a woman's milk after extreme exercise to cause babies to refuse the breast (Wallace, Inbar, and Ernsthausen 1992). Subsequent studies have found this not to be an issue (see [Mohrbacher 2010] for a review of this research). A large study from Australia found that exercise during the first postpartum year had no negative effect on breastfeeding initiation or duration (Su et al. 2007). Breastfeeding mothers do not need to restrict their exercise. You can exercise alone or find an exercise that you and your baby can do together: mom and baby exercise class, walking with the baby in a stroller or carrier, and walking or running with a jogging stroller are several options.

PERMS, HAIR DYES, TANNING BEDS, AND PIERCINGS

Using hair dye and getting permanents are also okay for breastfeeding mothers. There is no evidence that hair-care products get into a mother's milk. Similarly, tanning beds do not have any impact on your milk. Regarding nipple piercing, women with pierced nipples have safely breastfed their babies, as long as the jewelry is removed before breastfeeding.

Expressing and Storing Milk

Expressing milk refers to removing it from your breasts, either manually or with a breast pump. Not all breastfeeding mothers need to express their milk. But for most women who breastfeed for any length of time, knowing how to express milk is a useful skill.

There are many reasons women express their milk. The following are the most common:

- *To stay comfortable.* This is most likely during the first week or so after birth, when a mother's breasts may feel full even after her baby breastfeeds. This may also be useful during weaning.

- *To provide milk for feedings and/or stimulate milk production.* These may be important when

  - a mother and her baby are separated at feeding times;

  - the baby is unable or unwilling to breastfeed;

  - the baby is not breastfeeding effectively;

  - a mother wants her partner or the baby's siblings to feed the baby or prefers to feed her milk by bottle in some situations;

  - a mother wants to increase her milk production by draining her breasts more often or more fully.

Methods of Milk Expression

In many parts of the world, women express their milk by hand. However, in the United States, women most commonly express milk with a breast pump. If you use a pump, you may find the following tips helpful.

GIVE YOURSELF TIME TO PRACTICE

If you are pumping, know that it takes time to get accustomed to a breast pump and become proficient with it. Even with ample milk production, some mothers find it difficult to express their milk, especially at first and even with a good pump. If you need to express your milk on a regular basis, be sure to give yourself enough time to learn to use your pump and to become used to its feel.

FIND THE RIGHT FIT

The better pump companies (Ameda and Medela) offer flanges with different-sized nipple tunnels. If your nipples are rubbing uncomfortably along the sides of the pump nipple tunnel, too much of the area around your nipple is rubbing and uncomfortable, or you're not getting good results, you may need a larger or smaller size.

Expressing to Store Milk

If you're pumping to store milk, the following basics may be of help.

TRY PUMPING IN THE MORNING

Most women get more milk in the morning than later in the day. A good time to pump is usually thirty to sixty minutes after a nursing and at least an hour before a breastfeeding. The worst time is right before breastfeeding.

ENHANCE YOUR MILK RELEASE

Removing milk with a pump is not like sucking liquid through a straw. With a straw, the stronger you suck, the more liquid you get. With the breast, strength of suction is not the most important factor in effective pumping (Mitoulas et al. 2002). The key to expressing milk is triggering the let-down, or milk release.

During milk release, the breast actively moves the milk toward the nipple where the baby or pump can access it. Muscles within the breast squeeze both to push the milk out and to make the ducts widen. Some mothers feel this as a tingling sensation in their breasts; others feel nothing. A milk release can be triggered by a certain touch at the breast, hearing another mother's baby cry, or even by thinking about your baby. Feelings of tension, anger, or frustration can block it. Without a milk release, a mother will only express the small amount of milk pooled around the nipple, which makes triggering milk release vital to successful pumping.

During breastfeeding, most mothers have several milk releases without even knowing it (Ramsay et al. 2004). When your baby is at the breast, all the familiar physical cues (softness, warmth) and your loving emotions release the hormones that trigger milk release.

When a mother puts a pump to her breasts, though, these normal baby cues are missing. For this reason, some mothers need a little extra help at first in triggering milk releases as they adjust to the new feel of the pump. This can also happen when a mother switches from one pump to another (even from one hospital-grade pump to another), because the feel of the pump is different.

If you need some help releasing your milk to the pump, experiment with the following suggestions and see which work for you. You may only need to use one or two for a short time until the feel of the pump becomes familiar.

- *Feelings*: Close your eyes, relax, and imagine your baby is breastfeeding. Breathe slowly and deeply and think about how much you love your baby.

- *Sight:* Look at your baby or, if away from your baby, look at her photo.

- *Hearing:* Listen to a recording of your baby cooing or crying. If you're away, call your baby's caregiver and check on her. Call someone you love who can relax and distract you.

- *Smell:* Smell an item of your baby's clothing or her blanket.

- *Touch:* Apply warm compresses or gently massage your breasts.

- *Taste*: Sip a favorite warm drink to relax you.

The bottom line is this: more milk releases mean more milk expressed.

HOW MUCH MILK TO EXPECT PER PUMPING

If you are pumping between regular feedings and exclusively breastfeeding (using no formula) and your baby is gaining well, expect to pump about half a feeding. If you are pumping at feeding time for a missed feeding, expect to pump a full feeding. (Feeding amount will vary depending on your baby's age, as described in this next section.)

DECIDING HOW MUCH MILK TO LEAVE FOR YOUR BABY

A baby's milk intake varies by age and, up to a point, by weight.

During the first week...	most babies who were born full term take no more than 1–2 oz. (30–60 ml) at a feeding.
By the second and third week...	on average, they take about 2–3 oz. (60–90 ml).
Once they reach about four to five weeks...	they are at their peak milk intake of about 25–35 oz. (750–1,050 ml) per day, and, as explained in chapter 6, the amount your baby needs per day will not change until she starts taking other foods, at which point the amount needed will decrease.

For a baby between one and six months old an average feeding is about 3–4 oz. (90–120 ml). Although a baby gets bigger and heavier from one to six months, her growth rate slows down during that time, so the amount of milk she needs stays the same. Knowing this can be a huge relief if you are trying to keep up with your baby after returning to work.

HANDLING AND STORING HUMAN MILK

You will no doubt notice that milk storage guidelines differ from book to book, and it may help you to know why. Although your milk will not spoil before the times listed below, the longer it is stored, the more nutritional value is lost. That's why some guidelines suggest shorter storage times. It is always good to use your milk as quickly as you can after expressing it. But if you should find some stored milk in the back of your refrigerator that has been sitting there for seven days, one thing is for sure—it will still be much better for your baby than formula, which doesn't provide any illness prevention. In fact, it's those antibodies—the living parts of your milk—that kill bacteria in your milk, making it hardier than formula. When in doubt, smell or taste your milk. Spoiled milk will smell spoiled.

Storage Time for Human Milk

(for full-term, healthy babies)

Freshly expressed human milk

Freezer	Refrigerator	Room temperature (< 79°F; 25°C)
3–4 months in a refrigerator/freezer (in a sealed container)	8 days (for mature milk)	12–24 hours (for colostrum [milk expressed birth to day 5])
6–12 months in a deep freeze (0°F; -19°C or lower)		4-6 hours (for mature milk)

Freshly expressed milk also can be kept at < 60°F (15°C)—for example, in an insulated bag with cooling elements frozen—for up to 24 hours.

Previously frozen human milk

Freezer	Refrigerator	Room temperature (< 79°F; 25°C)
Do not refreeze.	24 hours	1 hour

Previously frozen human milk is best thawed under warm running water.

There is no research indicating whether the leftover portion of human milk that has been freshly expressed and then warmed should be discarded or saved.

These guidelines mean you can store freshly expressed milk at room temperature for four to six hours, then move it to the refrigerator for eight days, and then still freeze it.

Store milk in small amounts and warm with low heat. You can store your milk in any clean, sealed container, but you'll want to avoid using thin bottle liners, which can split when frozen. Store your milk in amounts no larger than you think your baby will take at one feeding. This will minimize waste and make it faster for you to warm it for a feeding. Having smaller amounts also allows you to give your baby more if she wants it. When warming milk, keep heat to a minimum, as high heat kills antibodies in the milk that keep your baby healthy. If your milk is frozen, thaw it in its container under cool then warmer running water until the milk is between room temperature and body temperature.

Milk layers and combining batches. Before you give your milk to your baby, gently swirl the container to mix the layers that have separated. (It is not homogenized like cow's milk from the store.) You can combine previously expressed milk with newly expressed milk if both are within the storage guidelines. Fresh cooled milk can be added to a container of frozen milk and then put back into the freezer as long as the amount of fresh milk is not greater than the amount of milk already frozen. When storing a combined batch of milk, date it according to the oldest milk. (For example, if refrigerated or frozen milk expressed on March 10 is combined with milk expressed on March 14, the new combined batch should be marked with a March 10 date.)

To freeze or not to freeze. If refrigerated milk will not be used within eight days, you'll need to freeze it. If you're storing milk prior to working outside the home, plan to freeze some milk for your first day back at work as well as some extra as a reserve. Once you start working, though, plan to give mostly fresh or refrigerated milk since freezing kills some of the antibodies in the milk that keep baby healthy. But even with fewer antibodies than fresh milk, it is still a huge improvement over formula.

Medications and Contraception

At some point while you're breastfeeding, you may need to take prescription or over-the-counter (OTC) medications. Most mothers do. According to Thomas Hale, R.Ph., Ph.D., author of *Medications and Mothers' Milk*, surveys indicate that between 90 and 99 percent of mothers take medications in their first week postpartum (Hale 2010).

What to Do If You Need to Take Medications

You might wonder if a medication prescribed for you could harm your breastfeeding baby. Some mothers are so fearful of this that they choose to wean their babies rather than risk exposure to the medication. This is a common reason women give for weaning their babies prematurely. However, weaning is almost always unnecessary. If you are taking medication, don't assume that your choice is between "contaminated" breast milk and "pristine" formula. According to the American Academy of Pediatrics, in the vast majority of cases, the risks of giving formula to your baby far outweigh the risks of continuing to breastfeed with a tiny bit of medication in your milk. And for most medications, your baby is only exposed to a very small amount of what you take (often less than 1 percent of your dose). There are very few medications that are not recommended for nursing mothers (Hale 2010).

Space does not permit us to list here all the medications that are compatible with breastfeeding. But there are two resources you might find helpful. The first is the American Academy of Pediatrics' publication *The Transfer of Drugs and Other Chemicals into Human Milk* (AAP 2001). This is available on our website (www.breastfeedingmade simple.com) for you to share with your doctor. The second resource is Thomas Hale's *Medications and Mothers' Milk* (Hale 2010). In the lactation field, this is considered the "bible" of drug use for nursing mothers. It is updated often and is relatively inexpensive. You might want to get a copy for yourself, especially if you frequently take medications. (See our Resources section for publication details and ordering information.) You can also call your local La Leche League leader or lactation consultant and ask them to look up any medications that you have questions about. Most have a copy of *Medications and Mothers'*

Milk and can answer your question. You might also want to check with Dr. Hale's Infant Risk Center for up-to-date information on medication use during pregnancy and breastfeeding (www.infantrisk.org).

WHEN YOUR DOCTOR TELLS YOU TO WEAN

If a health care provider recommends weaning because you are taking a medication, chances are weaning isn't necessary. If your doctor is relying on the *Physicians' Desk Reference* (PDR staff 2010), you should know that the information about breastfeeding provided there is often inaccurate. Drug manufacturers compile the PDR, and they are often more concerned about possible legal action (hence, the caution about advising breastfeeding moms not to use many medications) than they are about giving unbiased information on drugs and breastfeeding.

In contrast, *Medications and Mothers' Milk* (Hale 2010) looks specifically at the characteristics of the medication, how your body processes it, and how much is detectable in infants whose mothers have taken it. In most cases, if there is any medication detectable in the infant's blood, it is far below what would be considered a *clinical dose* (that is, a dose big enough to have any impact). Sharing this information with your baby's doctor is often enough to reassure her that the medication is compatible with breastfeeding. It's always in your best interest to be open with your health care providers about medications that you're taking (including OTC, herbal, and prescription medications) and to tell them that you are breastfeeding when any drugs are prescribed for you. Also, be aware of the possibility that something you are taking may interact with something that your baby is taking. The safest course is to tell your health care providers about everything both you and your baby take. You can also consult the Infant Risk Center for more detailed information (www.infantrisk.org).

SOME GENERAL GUIDELINES ON MEDICATION USE

Even though most medications are compatible with breastfeeding, you want to be sensible in their use. Here are some of Thomas Hale's (2010) general guidelines:

- *The smallest dose is best.* It's in your and your baby's best interest to use the smallest therapeutic dose that will help you. Take only the amount prescribed.

- *Your baby's age, weight, and the number of times she breast-feeds all make a difference.* Babies who are older, heavier, or who eat other foods (meaning that they breastfeed less) have less exposure to medications than babies who are premature, ill, small, or exclusively breastfeeding. However, even in the case of small or young babies, the exposure to medication is almost always less risky than weaning.

- *Drugs given to babies are usually okay for mothers to take.* If a medication is normally prescribed for infants to take (for example, amoxicillin), then it is generally appropriate for breastfeeding mothers to take. However, don't assume that a drug you took while pregnant is automatically fine for you to take while breastfeeding. It may be. But the way medications transfer to the baby during pregnancy (via your placenta) versus during breastfeeding (via your milk) can influence how much medication your baby is exposed to. It's always good to double-check.

HERBAL MEDICATIONS

In the past decade, complementary and alternative medications, in general, and herbal medicine, in particular, have become mainstream. Some health care providers are not terribly pleased about that. There are a number of advantages of herbs over traditional pharmaceutical medications, such as lower costs (especially for someone without prescription coverage), easier access, and fewer side effects. All of these factors are important and may be why you are considering taking herbs. Unfortunately, people often avoid telling their health care providers that they are taking herbs for fear that their providers will judge them. We can understand why this happens, but it is a dangerous practice in general and particularly now that you are breastfeeding. Patients have been so reticent about telling their doctors that they are taking herbs that the U.S. National Center for Complementary and

Alternative Medicine (NCCAM) has launched an "Ask, Tell" campaign to encourage doctors and patients to talk to each other.

We need to caution you that just because something is "natural" doesn't mean you should be careless in its use. Herbs are drugs, just like their pharmacologic counterparts. You should only take them if you have a specific need. Your safest course is to work with a licensed herbalist or other health care provider who is knowledgeable about herbs.

There are three good sources of information on the compatibility of herbs with breastfeeding: *Nursing Mother's Herbal* by Sheila Humphrey (2003), *The Complete German Commission E Monographs* (Blumenthal et al. 1998), and *Medications and Mothers' Milk* by Thomas Hale (2010). For information on where to find them, see References at the end of this book or our website (www.breastfeedingmadesimple.com).

Supplements

Since the first edition of this book came out, new guidelines have been released regarding two supplements recommended for pregnant and breastfeeding women: vitamin D and omega-3 fatty acids. At first, we were somewhat skeptical about the need for these. But we have become convinced after reviewing the research studies that have come out over the past five years.

VITAMIN D

Vitamin D has become a hot topic in perinatal health during the last ten years. Health care providers' interest in this vitamin increased when some children in North Carolina were identified as having rickets. Rickets is a disease of vitamin D deficiency, and it was thought to have been eradicated in developed countries. However, there have been some cultural and lifestyle issues that have led to its increased presence. First has been the recommendation to limit sun exposure due to realistic concerns about skin cancer. Exposure to the sun is necessary for our bodies to synthesize vitamin D, and avoiding the sun has led to the unintended consequence of vitamin D deficiency.

Second, our lifestyles now keep us inside more than we are outside, further limiting our sun exposure.

Unfortunately, rickets is not the only health problem associated with vitamin D deficiency. Vitamin D deficiency increases the risk of autoimmune disease, depression, and even cancer (Wagner, with Taylor and Hollis 2010). Furthermore, many women in developed countries are deficient, perhaps not to the point of having rickets, but under the levels they should be. This ongoing deficiency has implications for their health and for babies' growth during pregnancy and postpartum.

Based on results from two large clinical trials, Dr. Carol Wagner and her colleagues at the Medical University of South Carolina recommend that pregnant and breastfeeding women supplement with 4,000 IU of vitamin D per day, which is many times greater than the current recommendation of 400 IU per day.

Dr. Wagner and colleagues also recommend that infants receive vitamin D supplements of 400 IU/day. That recommendation is still somewhat controversial. But there is a concern that simply supplementing mothers is not enough to bring babies' levels to where they need to be (Wagner, with Taylor and Hollis 2010). There is currently a clinical trial underway that will provide more answers on this issue.

Our recommendation to you is that at the very least, make sure that *you* are not deficient. Your levels of vitamin D influence the amount of vitamin D your baby gets in your milk. Your adequate level of vitamin D may not be enough to keep your infant from being deficient. But your deficiency will only compound the problem. Talk with your health care provider about it. We also recommend the book, *New Insights into Vitamin D During Pregnancy, Lactation and Early Infancy* (Wagner, with Taylor and Hollis 2010), which is written for health care providers and includes a great summary of the current research and the rationale for supplementation of both mothers and infants.

OMEGA-3 FATTY ACIDS: EPA AND DHA

Mothers are also often deficient in the long-chain omega-3 fatty acids, EPA and DHA. This is a concern because these fatty acids (especially DHA) are essential for the growth and development of babies' vision and brain. The most common dietary source for EPA and DHA is fish. In cultures where women do not eat a lot of fish, they tend to be deficient, especially during pregnancy and postpartum. For example, speaking about mothers in Australia, Rees and colleagues noted that babies need about 67 mg per day of DHA during pregnancy for their developing nervous systems, while Australian mothers consume about 15 mg per day, well under what babies need (Rees, Austin, and Parker 2005). Because DHA is essential for babies to have, mothers' bodies will divert whatever stores the mothers have to their babies, meaning that mothers become more deficient with each pregnancy.

There is currently a lot of hype about formula companies adding DHA to infant formula. The brain-growth element has really been emphasized, with campaigns showing babies wearing mortarboards or working on the computer. These ads imply that if babies get these fatty acids in formula, they will become über-babies. That simply isn't the case. Supplementing to correct a deficiency means that babies will attain their normal level of intelligence. Giving a baby more DHA than they need will not increase their intelligence above this. Human milk, which also contains DHA, will always be vastly superior to formula no matter what they put in it.

We have another reason for recommending omega-3 supplementation: *your* health and well-being. There have been a number of research studies showing that fish consumption is related to lower rates of depression and other mental illnesses (see Kendall-Tackett, forthcoming, for a full review of these studies). In a study that specifically compared rates of postpartum depression with national rates of fish consumption, Joseph Hibbeln of the U.S. National Institutes of Health found that postpartum depression was up to twenty-five times more likely in countries that have low fish consumption (Hibbeln 2002). EPA and DHA also have the added benefit of decreasing stress—another way that they can benefit postpartum women.

Even though most of the studies have examined fish consumption, there are some problems with recommending that mothers eat a lot of fish because of contaminants in seafood. There is no way for consumers to know if fish is contaminated. The safest course is using fish-oil supplements. The U.S. Pharmacopeia tests brands of fish-oil products for contaminants and verifies specific brands as being contaminant free (these are listed on their website: www.USP.org). There are also vegetarian DHA products, but as of this writing, no vegetarian EPA. Flaxseed and other plant sources of omega-3s contain ALA, the parent omega-3 fatty acid. ALA is metabolically too far removed from EPA and DHA to have an antidepressant or antistress effect.

The current recommended dosages are 200–400 mg/day of DHA. This is the minimum, but it is likely on the low side. One recent article recommends 800–1,000 mg/day in order to decrease risk of depression (McNamara 2009). And this amount is in line with the amount of DHA women get in countries where people eat a lot of fish, such as Japan or Norway, where people consume 1,000 mg of DHA per day. For EPA, the amount to use for treating depression is 1,000 mg/day. EPA is often used in combination with DHA, or sometimes used alongside medications to make the medications more effective. In fact, the American Psychiatric Association (APA) considers EPA a promising treatment for mood disorders and recognizes its mental health benefits when used alone or in combination with medications (Freeman et al. 2006).

Note: As always, before taking any supplement, be sure to talk it over with your health care provider. We have also provided more information about omega-3s and breastfeeding on www.breastfeeding madesimple.com.

Contraception

Your choice of contraception may have an impact on breastfeeding, but most methods do not. Here is a brief summary of what you need to know.

CONTRACEPTION WITH NO EFFECT ON BREASTFEEDING

If you live in an industrialized country, you may be surprised to learn that breastfeeding itself is contraceptive—if breastfeeding meets certain criteria.

Lactation as contraception. Breastfeeding as contraception (called the *lactation amenorrhea method* or LAM) is most effective if a mother's periods have not returned and if the baby is

- not receiving other liquids or solids;

- not going longer than four hours between breastfeedings during the day and six hours at night;

- younger than six months old.

If a mother's periods have returned, she is supplementing, or she is going longer between feedings, her risk of pregnancy is increased. This explains why we all know of women who have gotten pregnant while breastfeeding. On the other hand, if a woman is exclusively breastfeeding (meaning that the baby receives no other liquids or solids), has not resumed menstruating, and meets the other criteria, the contraceptive effect of breastfeeding is around 98 percent.

Natural family planning. Another nonhormonal form of birth control is natural family planning (NFP). NFP teaches women to observe their body signs, such as changes in temperature, cervical mucus, and in the opening of the cervix, to determine times when she is fertile. She can then plan the timing of intercourse appropriately. Training is necessary for women to learn their fertility signals.

Barrier methods. Barrier methods, such as condoms, diaphragms, contraceptive sponges, or cervical caps, are also effective and relatively inexpensive and have no impact on breastfeeding. If spermicides are used, these are considered compatible with breastfeeding (Mohrbacher 2010).

Nonhormonal IUDs. Nonhormonal intrauterine devices (IUDs) are another possible method with no impact on breastfeeding. It is best if you have it inserted within two to four days after birth, or after six weeks postpartum.

Surgical sterilization. Tubal ligation is another method of contraception with no impact on breastfeeding. However, if you choose to have surgery immediately after birth, you will be separated from your baby, which will affect your ability to breastfeed frequently in the early days. You might consider delaying this procedure until breastfeeding is well established. A hysterectomy (full or partial, even with removal of the ovaries) will not affect breastfeeding.

HORMONAL METHODS OF CONTRACEPTION

Because the artificial hormones in hormonal birth control sometimes affect milk production, they are not the first choice for breastfeeding mothers. However, hormonal methods that use progestin only are considered compatible with breastfeeding (AAP 2001). Progestin-only methods include the minipill, progestin-IUDs, progestin-releasing vaginal rings, injectable contraceptives (such as Depo-Provera), and contraceptive implants (such as Norplant). Avoid these methods until you are at least six to eight weeks postpartum (Mohrbacher 2010).

Hormonal contraceptives with estrogen are not your best choice because estrogen can lower your milk production—in some cases, dramatically. If you decide to use an estrogen-based contraceptive, current recommendations are that you wait until your baby is at least six months old and eating other foods.

CHAPTER 10

Common Breastfeeding Challenges

Breastfeeding is a learned skill, and it can take time for it to feel natural. As you learn, you may encounter some challenges along the way. These challenges can be discouraging, but most can be overcome. In this chapter we offer some suggestions for dealing with the bumps in the road you and your baby might encounter.

Mother-Related Challenges

As we described in the first seven chapters, most of these challenges can be avoided by following the laws. But sometimes, even with the best intentions, life interferes and problems arise.

Engorgement

Engorgement in the early postpartum period occurs when increasing circulation, growing milk production, and retained tissue fluid "balloon" the breast beyond its comfortable capacity, according to Jean Cotterman, RNC, IBCLC. In its extreme forms, engorgement can be almost unbearably painful, and it may feel as though your breasts are going to burst. Engorgement can make the areola firm, making a deep latch difficult and sometimes causing the nipple to flatten. The areola must be soft enough to change shape during suckling, to let the nipple extend deep into the baby's mouth. When the breast becomes too firm, your baby may be unable to achieve this deep latch, putting you at risk for nipple pain and preventing the baby's tongue and jaws from pressing effectively on milk ducts within the breast.

WHAT YOU CAN DO

There are several things you can do to get you over this hurdle.

Drain your breasts frequently and well. Breastfeed your baby at least eight to twelve times a day. Try to breastfeed at least every hour and a half to two hours during the day and every two to three hours at night until engorgement has subsided. Make sure that your baby has a good latch and that you're in the comfort zone (see chapter 3). If your baby is not breastfeeding or not breastfeeding well, use a rental pump to drain your breasts well and often. Removing milk from your breasts relieves the congestion and helps the engorgement subside more quickly.

Avoid bottles, pacifiers, or supplements. Keep your baby at the breast for all suckling. However, if your baby is not breastfeeding well, he obviously still needs to be fed. The best milk to use is your own given in a cup, spoon, syringe, or bottle. See chapter 11 for more on feeding methods.

Relieve pressure. When you are engorged, your baby may not be able to latch on well. If that is the case, you have a few options, including Reverse Pressure Softening, breast compression while baby breastfeeds (see "Sleepy Baby" below), hand expression, and gentle pumping. *Reverse Pressure Softening* (RPS), a simple technique developed by Jean Cotterman, RNC, IBCLC, is a way to temporarily soften the areola (pigmented area around the nipple), making latching and milk removal easier by moving some swelling slightly backward and upward into the breast. (For full instructions and line drawings, see our website, www. breastfeedingmadesimple.com.)

Use warmth. Warm compresses before you breastfeed can help the milk flow. Only use warmth right before breastfeeding since heat can increase inflammation.

Use cold. At other times, try cold. You can use an ice pack with crushed ice, a reusable soft ice pack, or a bag of frozen peas or corn. Wrap cold compresses in a towel to protect your skin and apply them for fifteen to twenty minutes at a time.

Wear a supportive bra. A sports bra or other supportive bra can be helpful. If it feels good, you can even wear one at night. Avoid underwire bras or those that are too tight, since consistent compression on the breast can cause mastitis.

Watch for possible infection. If your temperature rises above 100.6°F (38.4°C) and/or you are having any symptoms that feel like the flu, call your health care provider. You may have an infection.

Take an anti-inflammatory. Ibuprofen or other anti-inflammatories can help with discomfort, and most are compatible with breastfeeding. Ask your health care provider to recommend one.

If you follow the above suggestions, your symptoms should clear in a day or two. If they do not, don't try to tough it out. Contact skilled breastfeeding help. There could be something else going on. And remember, this too shall pass.

Nipple Pain and Trauma

Nipple pain can be very discouraging and can even make you depressed! The good news is that it should not hurt to breastfeed. More than a twinge at the beginning during the first week or two means that an adjustment is needed. And this isn't an invitation to beat yourself up for not breastfeeding perfectly. It's just a reminder to get the help you need to make breastfeeding comfortable for you.

NIPPLE TRAUMA IS NOT NORMAL

One pervasive idea that we'd love to change is that nipple trauma is normal during breastfeeding, a common cultural belief that has undermined breastfeeding for countless mothers. Although many mothers experience some discomfort during breastfeeding at first, the only type of nipple pain that we consider normal today is very mild tenderness at the beginning of a feeding during the first week or two after birth. Nipple discomfort that is truly in this normal range subsides after a minute or two of breastfeeding, when the mother's milk is released or lets down, and is not excruciating.

Many mothers have pain well outside these normal parameters but mistakenly believe or, unfortunately, are sometimes explicitly told that they have to endure it until it goes away on its own. They may delay seeking help or even give up on breastfeeding entirely. And honestly, we can't blame them. Pain during breastfeeding is a common reason women wean before they had planned to.

Note: Nipple pain is not "normal" when it includes any of the following:

- intense, toe-curling pain

- pain throughout the feeding or between feedings

- broken skin, blisters, or color changes

- a burning sensation during, after, or in between feedings

- persistent soreness that does not improve after a day or two of trying to correct the problem

Any woman experiencing any of these should seek skilled breastfeeding help immediately. And if you are still experiencing pain, and a health care provider tells you that your latch looks "fine," please get a second (or third or fourth) opinion. Your latch may look "fine," but if you are experiencing pain, there is likely something else going on.

Following are some of the more common causes of nipple pain and what you can do about them.

SHALLOW LATCH

Shallow latch is one of the most common causes of nipple pain. Some of the telltale signs are

- a nipple that emerges from your baby's mouth oddly shaped, with its surface at an angle, like a new tube of lipstick;

- a vertical or horizontal crease on your nipple, or a scab that develops on the face of the nipple.

Shallow latch can be caused or aggravated by engorgement or the use of bottles and pacifiers. Unusual anatomy in mother or baby, such as tongue-tie or inverted nipples, and "fit" issues will be covered later in this chapter and in chapter 11. For any problem with latch, review chapter 3 for suggestions on how to improve it.

When using laid-back breastfeeding positions, one way to improve a painful latch is to pull out your baby's lower lip if he has sucked it in.

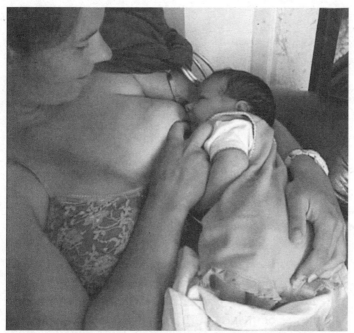

If breastfeeding hurts and your baby has her lower lip sucked in, pull her lip out. (©2010 Suzanne Colson, used with permission)

OTHER CAUSES OF NIPPLE PAIN

Nipple pain can also be due to other problems.

Not breaking baby's suction. You can cause nipple trauma by taking your baby off your breast without first releasing the suction in his mouth. We always wince when we see moms do this. Moms of older babies sometimes find that their nipples are sore because babies turn their heads to see what is going on while still attached to Mom—ouch! To remove the baby safely, slide your little finger into the corner of your baby's mouth between his gums until he releases your breast. Then remove your breast from his mouth.

Improper use of a breast pump. A wide variety of breast pumps are on the market. Some are excellent; others are not. Some of the discount pumps can be too strong and can damage your nipples. Also, some mothers mistakenly believe that if they crank their pump to the maximum setting, it will give them even more milk. This doesn't help. A too-tight fit can cause pain, too. Never continue to use a pump if it hurts.

Cleaning products and personal-care practices. Sometimes moms get sore nipples because of overzealous cleaning. You don't need to clean your breasts before you breastfeed. Your body already does this for you. If you use a topical ointment, choose one that does not need to be wiped off before your baby breastfeeds (such as Lansinoh ultra-purified lanolin, as described below). Also avoid breast pads or bras with plastic liners as these can trap moisture next to the nipple and cause skin breakdown.

Raynaud's phenomenon. Raynaud's phenomenon involves an involuntary constriction of the arteries so that body parts (usually hands or feet) blanch or turn white, blue, and/or red. This can also happen in the nipples, and it can cause searing nipple pain. If your nipple blanches after you nurse, ask a lactation consultant or your health care provider to evaluate it. If necessary, the prescription drug nifedipine, a beta blocker, can sometimes be helpful with Raynaud's and is compatible with breastfeeding. Raynaud's phenomenon is a common symptom of autoimmune disease, but it can also occur by itself.

Infections of the breast and skin problems. Infections can also cause severe pain. These can include mastitis and thrush (a yeast infection) and bacterial infections of the skin, as well as skin problems such as contact dermatitis, eczema, and psoriasis. These are described in more detail below.

Nipple bleb. This is a white spot on the nipple that sometimes causes pain during breastfeeding. Possible causes include a plugged milk duct or skin blocking the milk duct. It sometimes develops after nipple trauma. A bleb may or may not be painful. If it doesn't hurt, no treatment is needed. If it hurts, apply wet heat before breastfeeding by soaking the nipple in either the bath or the sink or by applying wet warm compresses. The idea is to thin the skin so that the baby can more easily draw out the plug of thickened milk during breastfeeding. If the bleb is not relieved with wet heat and breastfeeding, try the following:

* Wear a cotton ball soaked with olive oil in your bra between feedings to soften the skin.

* Once the skin is softened, try to peel away any thickened skin over the bleb and then try to manually express the plug.

If these do not provide relief, ask your health care provider to open the bleb. Immediate milk flow should bring relief. If the bleb is dry and the milk doesn't flow, continue trying the above.

If blebs recur, try eliminating saturated fats from your diet and taking lecithin supplements (one tablespoon three times per day or one to two 1,200 mg capsules three or four times per day).

WHAT YOU CAN DO

You don't have to keep suffering in order to breastfeed your baby. There are a variety of things that you can do to eliminate nipple pain. You will need to continue to drain your breasts, either by breastfeeding or by pumping. Don't wean suddenly, as you will likely end up with a worse problem (see chapter 7).

Make sure that your baby is latching deeply. Toughing it out does no one any good. If things don't seem to be any better within a day or so, contact skilled breastfeeding help and arrange to see someone.

Offer your least sore breast first. If you have nipple trauma, try different breastfeeding positions to find one that doesn't hurt or put pressure on any tender spots until help arrives. You might also try offering your less sore breast first and then switch to the other side after your milk lets down.

Express your milk. If your nipples are severely damaged or infected, you may prefer to rent a pump to drain your breasts until things heal up a bit. Don't use a cheap pump, or things might get worse. Some mothers find that pumping hurts less than breastfeeding. Just remember that you will need to drain your breasts at least eight times a day.

Use ultrapurified lanolin (such as Lansinoh brand) if you have trauma. It is no longer recommended to keep broken skin on your nipple dry. Lanolin provides moist wound healing, allowing your nipple to heal without forming a scab. Creating a healthy moisture balance reduces pain and speeds healing. If the friction of your clothing bothers you, use Lansinoh with breast shells (hard plastic shells worn in your bra) to prevent clothing friction on your nipples. If you use breast shells, be sure your bra cup is large enough to accommodate them without putting pressure on your breasts.

Use hydrogel pads. A new treatment for nipple pain and trauma is hydrogel dressings (one example is the Ameda ComfortGels), a soothing gel pad worn in the bra that also provides moist wound healing to reduce pain and speed healing. In a study, hydrogel dressings decreased women's pain more than lanolin without increasing the risk of infection (Dodd and Chalmers 2003). Ask your lactation consultant or hospital about them.

Treat infections or skin problems. If you have a bacterial or fungal infection (see below), see your practitioner about treatment. You can continue to breastfeed while you are being treated for an infection, but in some cases (as with thrush), your baby may need to be treated, too.

Mastitis

Mastitis refers to any inflammation of the breast, with or without a fever. A mild form of mastitis—a tender spot or lump in your breast with no fever—is sometimes referred to as a plugged or blocked duct.

If you have a temperature of more than 101°F (38.4°C), are achy, or have other symptoms that feel like the flu, you most likely have a more severe case that has progressed into an infection. Other signs of infection include a cracked nipple with pus, pus or blood in your milk, red streaks on your breast, and symptoms that appear suddenly and are severe.

WHAT YOU CAN DO

For mastitis with and without infection, the treatment is generally the same. However, if you think you have an infection, call your health care provider and ask about a prescription of antibiotics and then follow the suggestions we describe below.

Breastfeed frequently on the affected breast. Let your baby drain the affected breast frequently and/or use a pump. Allowing milk to accumulate in your breast will make matters worse. You may hesitate to breastfeed because it is uncomfortable. If so, try different positions until you find the one that is most comfortable. You might also talk with your health care provider about using an over-the-counter medication, such as ibuprofen, to lessen your symptoms and to help with pain. If your baby refuses to nurse on your affected side, you may need to pump on that side until the infection heals.

Apply heat to the area and gently massage it. Massage the area with your palm and fingers in a circular motion. You can also use your fingertips to knead your breast. Move from your armpit to your nipple. You can also soak your breast in warm water in a bath or leaning over a basin. Do this at least three times a day.

Breastfeed your baby immediately after you treat with heat. This will help loosen the plug.

Wear loose clothing. Avoid tight or restrictive clothing while healing mastitis. Also consider whether your bra is too tight. A tight bra can actually cause mastitis.

Rest. Mastitis may be your body's way of telling you that you are doing too much. Be sure to rest as much as you can to allow your body's natural defenses to fight any possible infection. Mothers who have recurrent cases of mastitis are often the ones who are running themselves ragged.

Consider possible causes. Your key to avoiding another case of mastitis may be to determine why you got it in the first place. Two common causes are broken skin on the nipple and a bra that's too tight. Another is anything that allows the breast to become overly full, such as irregular feeding patterns, a sudden change (such as when your baby begins sleeping through the night), the use of supplements, bottles, or a pacifier, or lengthening the times between feedings. Too-full breasts can also happen at times when you're really busy and go longer between feedings (holidays and family get-togethers can be key times). If any of these situations apply to you, do what you can to change them to help avoid a recurrence of your symptoms. And remember, sudden weaning can make matters worse.

Thrush or Yeast Infections

Another type of possible infection is caused by yeast (*Candida albicans*). Yeast infections can be painful for both mothers and babies. Your baby can have a yeast infection, which will appear as white patches inside his mouth (thrush) or as diaper rash.

Your baby may have a yeast infection if he has diaper rash, discomfort in his mouth at feedings, white patches in his mouth, or a white tongue (he does not have to have all of these symptoms). You may have a yeast infection if you have nipple pain that is burning or shooting (rather than stabbing or pinching, as from other causes). You may have redness, scaling, or flaking; the skin of the areola may be smooth and shiny; or your breasts may not look different at all. The pain may begin after a period of pain-free breastfeeding and may be quite severe.

Your nipples may or may not be itchy. It may be worse after feeding or at night. *Candida albicans* can cause nipple pain even if no thrush is seen in baby's mouth.

If you have a yeast infection on your nipples, it's important for you to treat both yourself and your baby. Yeast is contagious. Unless you both are treated, you are likely to reinfect each other. You may also need to treat any other family members (including your partner) if they have symptoms of yeast.

WHAT YOU CAN DO

The following are treatment options for your baby; work with your health care provider to find the best medication for you to use. Treatments for your baby include nystatin suspension (which has become much less effective in recent years due to its common usage, leading to the spread of nystatin-resistant strains of thrush), gentian violet, clotrimazole, and fluconazole.

Treatment options for you include the following:

- nystatin cream or ointment

- gentian violet

- over-the-counter antifungal creams such as

  - clotrimazole (sold as Mycelex, Lotrimin, Lotrimin AF cream or lotion [1 percent])

  - miconazole (sold as Mycatin, Monistat-Derm cream or lotion [2 percent])

  - ketoconazole (sold as Nizoral)

- nystatin with triamcinolone (a corticosteroid)

- Dr. Jack Newman's All Purpose Nipple Ointment (a prescribed option)

For more specific information, see our website (www.breastfeeding madesimple.com).

If you have deep breast pain, it may or may not be due to yeast. More commonly, deep breast pain is due to a bacterial infection of the nipple or Raynaud's phenomenon (see "Other Causes of Nipple Pain," above). Contact your health care provider or lactation specialist for further help.

Low Milk Production

Being worried about low milk production is the most common reason mothers give for premature weaning. Sometimes, a mother's milk production is not low at all. She only thinks it is. If you are not sure, review chapters 4 and 5. These will give you some specific guidelines on what is normal and how to tell whether your baby is getting enough milk.

WHAT YOU CAN DO

If after reviewing these chapters you decide that you need to increase your milk production—or if your baby has been losing or not gaining weight—here are some techniques to help you make more milk.

Breastfeed more. Try to feed at least eight to twelve times per day, and drain the breasts more fully each time. As we described in chapter 6, the more times per day that milk is effectively removed, the faster your milk production will increase. Focus on the number of feedings per day, not the time between feedings (for example, every two or three hours). Encourage the baby to breastfeed whenever he shows feeding cues, such as rooting, hand to mouth, or fussing, even if it has only been a short time since he last ate. To drain more milk each time, use each breast more than once and express milk after feedings.

Work to improve baby's latch. Review chapter 3 to help improve the baby's latch. A deeper latch will help your baby remove more milk from your breast, thereby signaling your body to make more.

Use breast compression. If your baby stops nursing actively or falls asleep within ten minutes at breast, stimulate baby to breastfeed actively for longer by using breast compression and by switching breasts (see "Sleepy Baby" later in this chapter).

Pump with a rental pump. *Double pump* (pump both breasts at the same time) for ten to fifteen minutes either right after feedings or after about half an hour. The more times per day the breasts are effectively drained, the more milk production is increased. Rental pumps are considered the most effective. If possible, pump long enough so that two minutes pass after you see the last drop of milk, or pump twenty to thirty minutes, whichever comes first. This has been found to increase milk production faster.

Decrease supplementation. If your baby is younger than one month, consider supplementing with a feeding method other than bottles, such as an at-breast supplementer, cup, syringe, or spoon (see chapter 11). Gradually decrease the supplementation as your milk production increases.

Try herbs or other medications to increase milk. The herb fenugreek is another way to increase your production. Fenugreek has a long history of use as a *galactagogue*, or substance that increases milk production, and the U.S. Food and Drug Administration has given it a rating of GRAS (generally recognized as safe). However, it can interact with a few prescription and over-the-counter medications and should be discussed with your health care provider before you take it (Hale 2010; Humphrey 2003). Take three to four capsules (of at least 500 mg each) three times per day (at least nine total per day). This is a higher dose than is on the label because label dosages are not for increasing milk. You can buy fenugreek at health food stores.

Two prescription medications that increase milk production are metoclopramide (Reglan) and domperidone (Motilium). Both are drugs normally prescribed for stomach problems. Studies indicate that metoclopramide and domperidone can increase milk production. Domperidone is currently under an FDA ban in the United States and is therefore not available at this writing. It is currently available in other countries, however, and is highly effective (see our website at www.breastfeeding madesimple.com for updated information). **Note:** Since depression can be a side effect of metoclopramide, you may want to avoid it if you have a history of depression (Hale 2010). Talk to your doctor about it.

There is also a rare side effect that happens most often with extended use of metoclopramide called *tardive dyskinesia*, or involuntary grimacing. Both of these side effects make metoclopramide a less-than-optimal choice. But it can be helpful in some circumstances. For more complete information on treatments for low milk production, we recommend *The Breastfeeding Mother's Guide to Making More Milk*, by Diana West and Lisa Marasco (2009).

Overabundant Milk Production

Mothers can also have too much milk. While this is a better problem to have than too little milk, it still can cause difficulties. Too much milk can be mighty unpleasant for your baby. To understand how he feels, think what it would be like for you if someone were to pour a quart of liquid into your mouth, giving you no way to control the flow. Overabundance can be why babies will sometimes push away from the breast, pull back, clamp down on the nipple, or refuse to breastfeed altogether. Some signs that indicate that you may have too much milk include the following:

- Your baby is gaining much more than 2 pounds (907 g) per month.

- He has trouble keeping up with the flow of your milk, and he gulps, chokes, or sputters when he nurses.

- He seems unusually gassy or has frothy or explosive stools.

This last point, in and of itself, does not indicate overabundant milk production, but when seen in combination with an unusually large weight gain, it may be another clue.

WHAT YOU CAN DO

Fortunately, there are some simple things that you can do to help your baby cope with your abundance of milk. The most straightforward technique is to limit each feeding session to only one breast. That decreases the overall amount of milk the baby receives. If needed, you can pump to comfort on the other side, but you don't want to completely drain your breast since this will signal your body to keep making lots of milk. Try this for four to seven days to see if your baby's symptoms improve.

Use one breast for more than one feeding. If your baby is still having difficulty coping with a forceful milk flow and is gaining much more weight than average, there are some other techniques that you can try. Use the same breast for two or three feedings in a row, pumping the other breast only to comfort as needed. If you have a very large over-production, this can help your body adjust more rapidly.

Try different positions. The laid-back breastfeeding positions described in chapters 1 and 3 are ideal, because gravity makes the milk flow more manageable. You might also find that the side-lying position works well for you because your baby can let milk dribble out of his mouth, rather than feeling like he needs to swallow to keep from choking.

Other options. You can also try starting the flow of your milk by hand expressing or using a pump. When the flow of milk has slowed somewhat, then put the baby to breast. Other mothers have found that a nipple shield (a flexible silicone nipple worn over your breast during feedings, used for a few days or weeks) can help babies cope with the flow of their mothers' milk. Frequent nursings can also help since less milk will have accumulated in the breast, making it easier for your baby to cope.

As a final caution, be sure that you never hold your baby's head to your breast to make sure that he breastfeeds. If your baby feels like he's choking, your holding his head there can make him not want to go anywhere near your breast, even when really hungry. Again, think how you would feel if someone were forcing a quart of liquid down your throat. If you allow your baby to have some control over how much milk he takes as he sucks and swallows, your baby's time at your breast will be much more pleasant for both of you.

Baby-Related Challenges

The following are some challenges that relate more to your baby than to you.

Sleepy Baby

Most newborns need to feed eight to twelve times per twenty-four hours to gain and grow well. But some babies don't know this and may need to be reminded to feed often enough and long enough. You will know you need to actively help your baby to feed more often or for a longer time if he

- has lost more than 10 percent of his birth weight in the first three to four days;

- is not gaining at least 5 oz. (140 g) per week after day four;

- is falling asleep before at least ten to fifteen minutes of good, active sucking on the first breast during the first week of life (this is not a problem if weight gain is good);

- has fewer than three to four good-sized stools per twenty-four hours (this is not a problem if weight gain is good);

- is jaundiced.

TO INCREASE THE NUMBER OF FEEDINGS

To increase the number of times your baby breastfeeds per day, you may need to help your baby take the breast more often. To do this, first make sure your baby is not swaddled and/or too warm. Swaddling suppresses your baby's feeding behaviors and as your baby gets warmer, sleepiness increases and active sucking decreases. Dress your baby in the same weight clothing that you would wear and even lighter when breastfeeding, as your body heat will warm him, too. Lean back and place your baby tummy down on your body in the laid-back positions illustrated in chapter 3. Wait until he is in a light sleep cycle. You'll know he's in a light sleep cycle if his eyes are moving under his eyelids or if his mouth or any other body part is moving. Babies pass in and out of deep sleep often. Just wait.

Trigger his inborn feeding behaviors and help him to the breast. Research from the United Kingdom found, amazingly, that newborns don't have to be awake to breastfeed effectively (Colson, DeRooy, and Hawdon 2003). In this study, mothers of late preterm babies were encouraged to keep their babies on their bodies in laid-back breastfeeding positions as much as possible during their first few days of life. These positions provided regular triggers for the babies' feeding behaviors. Mothers also stimulated feedings by stroking their babies or moving them to the breast while they were in a light sleep. Without completely waking, the babies responded by taking the breast and breastfeeding actively. Just like these mothers, if you help your baby to the breast when he's in a light sleep, you can increase the number of daily feedings without even having to awaken your baby.

TO INCREASE THE LENGTH OF FEEDINGS

Increasing the number of feedings will not help if the baby falls asleep at the breast before getting enough milk. Here are some techniques to help increase the amount of time babies spend breastfeeding actively.

Work to improve baby's latch. Getting the nipple into the comfort zone will ensure that your baby gets a faster milk flow to keep him more interested (see chapter 3).

Breast compression. This technique was popularized by pediatrician Jack Newman, MD. It increases the flow of milk to the baby, keeping him interested and feeding actively for longer. Leave your baby on the first breast to "finish" before switching breasts. As Dr. Newman writes: "How do you know the baby is finished? When he no longer drinks at the breast" (Newman and Pitman 2006, 72–73).

Follow these steps to do breast compression:

1. If you're in a sitting position, hold the baby with one arm and hold your breast with the opposite hand. If you're laid-back, hold your breast with a free hand.

2. Position your thumb on one side of the breast and your other fingers on the other side, well away from the nipple and areola (the dark area around your nipple).

3. Watch for the wide jaw movements that tell you your baby is getting milk. The baby gets more milk when he is drinking with an open mouth wide–pause–close mouth type of suck. (The "open mouth wide–pause–close mouth" sequence is one suck; the pause is not a pause between sucks.)

4. When the baby is nibbling or no longer drinking with the open mouth wide–pause–close mouth type of suck, compress the breast. Don't compress so hard that it hurts, and try not to change the shape of the breast near the baby's mouth. With the compression, the baby should start drinking again with the open mouth wide–pause–close mouth type of suck.

5. Keep the pressure up (don't stop compressing) until the baby is no longer drinking milk actively even with the compression, then release the pressure. Often the baby will stop sucking when the pressure is released but will start again shortly as milk starts to flow. If the baby does not stop sucking with the release of pressure, wait a short time before compressing again.

6. The reason to release the pressure is to allow your hand to rest and to allow milk to start flowing to the baby again. The baby, if he stops sucking when you release the pressure, will start again when he starts to taste milk.

7. When the baby starts sucking again, he may drink (open mouth wide–pause–close mouth). If not, compress again as above.

8. Continue on the first side until the baby does not drink, even with the compression. You should allow the baby to stay on

this side for a short time longer, as you may occasionally get another milk release and the baby will start drinking again on his own. If the baby no longer drinks, however, allow him to come off or take him off the breast. Breast compression is usually not needed for more than a few days if it is done consistently at every feeding. The baby will learn to stay active without help, although some pauses are always normal (Newman and Pitman 2006).

Switch breasts. When breast compression no longer works to keep your baby active, break the suction and take your baby off the breast. Change his diaper or stimulate him by stroking or undressing him even more, then offer the other breast. Repeat as many times as needed until baby is done.

Other options. There are a few other things that you can try to encourage more breastfeeding. You can try different breastfeeding positions, rub your baby's feet, undress him, or change his diaper. Once your baby starts taking more milk, he will perk up and these techniques won't be necessary.

Exaggerated Newborn Jaundice

Babies are born with extra red blood cells. These extra cells break down in the early weeks of life, producing a substance called bilirubin. When there is too much bilirubin in your baby's blood, he becomes jaundiced and his skin takes on a yellow hue. Jaundice is a common condition, occurring in more than half of all newborns (Mohrbacher 2010). Although this puts newborn jaundice in the "normal" category, jaundice is important for your baby's doctor to monitor since it can lead to more serious conditions if it becomes severe.

Finding out that your baby has exaggerated jaundice can be frightening. And sometimes the steps taken to correct it can interfere with breastfeeding. The standard advice used to be that mothers should stop breastfeeding so their babies could be treated. However, research has revealed that breastfeeding actually helps resolve jaundice. So in most cases, you should continue breastfeeding without interruption.

DIFFERENT TYPES OF JAUNDICE

There are different types of jaundice, and some require no treatment. One way that doctors tell the difference between the types of jaundice is by the timing of the first symptoms. If the jaundice appears on the first day, it generally indicates a physical cause unrelated to feeding, such as Rh and ABO blood compatibilities, liver enzyme deficiency diseases, or conditions such as gastrointestinal obstructions. With rare exceptions, breastfeeding should proceed normally.

Jaundice that appears on days two to five is more common, occurring in about half of all newborns. Some babies, such as those of Asian, Native American/American Indian, or South American ethnicity normally have higher levels of bilirubin. Unless baby's bilirubin reaches unsafe levels, normal newborn jaundice tends to resolve on its own within a few days or weeks, especially if the baby is feeding eight to twelve times in twenty-four hours and is passing stools. Indeed, effective breastfeeding (at least nine to eleven times per day from birth in one study) prevents exaggerated bilirubin levels (levels higher than 15 mg/dl; Yamauchi and Yamanouchi 1990).

Colostrum, the early milk, also acts as a natural laxative and helps the baby eliminate bilirubin through his stools. If babies don't receive enough colostrum in the first few days, the meconium, the black tarry stool, may not be passed, and the bilirubin in the meconium will be reabsorbed into their bloodstreams (causing bilirubin levels to rise). Babies at risk for exaggerated jaundice are those who are not feeding well. Those at higher risk are babies born *late-preterm* (thirty-four to thirty-seven weeks gestation), who are often sent home from the hospital not feeding well. Exaggerated newborn jaundice is one common reason for these babies to be readmitted to the hospital.

Jaundice can even appear after the baby's first week. There is a condition called *late-onset* or *breast-milk* jaundice that researchers are discovering may be more common than previously believed. It may affect up to one-third of babies. Indeed, researchers are beginning to speculate that this might be the normal pattern, rather than the abnormally low level of bilirubin found in formula-fed babies. As long as bilirubin levels are not in the unhealthy range (generally above 20 mg/dl), this condition will generally resolve on its own without treatment.

258

One difficulty of jaundice is that it tends to make babies sleepy. Moms sometimes don't realize that anything is amiss, only that their babies seem to sleep a lot. Unfortunately, these babies are often the ones who are not feeding well simply because they are not breastfeeding enough times during the day. Moreover, these babies may fall asleep at the breast before they've had enough milk. The result is poor weight gain and bilirubin levels that are too high. See the suggestions in the "Sleepy Baby" section, above, for coaxing a sleepy baby to eat.

TREATMENTS FOR JAUNDICE

Fortunately for mothers and babies, strategies recommended for jaundice have changed in recent years to encourage breastfeeding. In most cases, as long as breastfeeding is going well, a mother should continue breastfeeding with health care providers checking baby's bilirubin level from time to time. Effective breastfeeding should guarantee the passage of many stools per day, which is the primary way baby clears the bilirubin from his system. You should also avoid giving water supplements to your baby since these slow the clearance of bilirubin by cutting down on the number of times that babies breastfeed and produce stools during the day.

In previous times, the standard protocol for treatment of jaundice was to use formula. Fortunately, this is no longer the case. However, there are some times when formula is called for. If your milk production is low, you may need to use formula for a few feedings to increase the number of stools that your baby has. However, while doing this, you can start pumping your breasts to increase your milk production. Any expressed milk that you have can be given to your baby.

Your doctor may want your baby to receive *phototherapy*, which may involve either placing the baby under lights or using a special wrap that helps break down bilirubin through the skin. If lights are used, your baby will be placed under them wearing only a diaper and some protective patches on his eyes. You may be able to rent phototherapy equipment to provide treatment at home. If your baby is rehospitalized, you may be able to stay in the nursery with your baby or have the *bililights* set up in your hospital room. When your baby seems hungry, you can remove him from the lights, breastfeed him, and then return him to the lights, as the lights do not need to be used continuously to be effective. With proper management, the jaundice should safely clear in a few days or weeks without compromising breastfeeding. See our website (www.breastfeedingmadesimple.com) for the American Academy of Pediatrics treatment guidelines that you can share with your baby's doctor.

Breast Refusal or Nursing Strike

A baby who refuses to breastfeed can be devastating for any mom. Your baby may refuse the breast as a newborn, or he may suddenly refuse to breastfeed after several weeks or months of breastfeeding well. This is called a *nursing strike*.

It's very easy to think that your baby doesn't like you or your milk, and your baby's behavior can feel like a personal rejection. If you are feeling that way, we can totally sympathize. However, we also want to reassure you that your baby is not making a judgment about you. It's true that your baby may not like breastfeeding—at the moment. But your baby prefers you to all other people. He recognizes the sound of your voice, the smell of your body, and the unique taste of your milk. Just smelling or hearing you reassures him. So what we need to focus on right now is how to make breastfeeding a more pleasurable experience for you both. Unfortunately, when you feel rejected, it takes you out of problem-solving mode. So we ask that, for the moment, you try to see this from the baby's perspective, which will often suggest a solution.

TRY TO LOCATE A CAUSE

When dealing with a nursing strike, locating the possible cause can be helpful. It would probably be a good time for you to call a lactation consultant or a mother-to-mother breastfeeding counselor in your area to see if the two of you can figure this out. If no one is available, we'll give you some suggestions about where to start.

Did your baby have an injury at birth or might he be in pain? Sometimes babies refuse the breast because they are uncomfortable when held in a certain position. If your baby's mouth was roughly suctioned at birth, he may have a sore throat or be afraid to allow anything into his mouth. If you suspect that this might be the case, try various positions to see if one is more comfortable for you and your baby. Try the hardwiring ideas in chapter 1 to help your baby feel more at ease when held close.

Do you have a forceful let-down? Earlier in this chapter, we discussed what happens when your baby is trying to cope with too much milk all at once. See "Overabundant Milk Production" earlier in this chapter for some suggestions about how to cope with this.

Have you or someone else been trying to force your baby to breastfeed? This can happen when well-meaning moms or helpers decide to force the baby to the breast. Your baby may get to the point where he wants nothing to do with it.

Does your baby have a deep latch? With a shallow latch, many babies are unable to stimulate a good milk flow. This can be frustrating for them. Review chapter 3 for suggestions.

Is your baby getting enough milk when he feeds? Sometimes breastfeeding, especially early on, is frustrating for babies when they are really hungry and there is little milk. If your production is low and/or your baby is very hungry, your baby may find that nursing isn't much fun.

Is your baby ill or has he been biting? A baby may refuse to breastfeed when he has an ear infection (which makes breastfeeding painful) or a cold. You may want to see your baby's health care provider to rule out a physical problem. If your baby has bitten you and you startled him by jumping or yelling (an understandable reaction!), that can sometimes cause a baby to temporarily refuse the breast.

Has something changed in your life? Babies sometimes react to a prolonged separation or unusual stress in the family by refusing the breast.

WHAT YOU CAN DO

Fortunately, there are some steps you can take to help coax your baby back onto the breast.

Have lots of contact with your baby. Review chapter 2 and have lots of skin-to-skin contact with your baby. Carry your baby. Sleep with him. Offer the breast when he's in a quiet, alert state, but not necessarily hungry. Make the breast a pleasant place to be.

Try breastfeeding when your baby is asleep or half asleep. If they are not fully awake, many babies will breastfeed without thinking.

Watch for early hunger cues. Mothers can have difficulties when they wait until their babies are frantically hungry before feeding them. As we described earlier, your baby will be a lot more cooperative if he is not famished.

Take advantage of your baby's hardwiring. See chapters 1 and 2 for ways to calm and relax your baby. Your baby is born wanting to breastfeed. Use his natural responses to help make it happen.

Feed the baby and protect your production. The refusal to nurse can take a few days to resolve. In the meantime, you need to protect your milk production and feed your baby. See chapter 11 for suggestions on preserving your milk production with a pump. You may also need to feed your baby either your pumped milk or some supplementary formula if your milk production is low. Just keep in mind that the goal is to return your baby happily to the breast.

Get help. Don't hesitate to get skilled breastfeeding help if you're not making progress on your own.

You and your baby can overcome breast refusal or a nursing strike. Get support and have patience. It's well worth the extra effort.

CHAPTER 11

Special Situations: Physical or Health Issues

Sometimes breastfeeding can be challenging because of illness or an ongoing physical issue. In this chapter, we describe some strategies you can use if you encounter difficulties in your own or your baby's health that are influencing breastfeeding. We'll also offer suggestions on what you can do.

Special Situations: Mother

Many mothers worry that breastfeeding may be compromised if they have an acute or chronic illness, if they are depressed or have other emotional issues, or if there is something unusual about their anatomy. That's what this section is about. We want you to know up front that there are few reasons to wean, even temporarily. In most cases, breastfeeding will still be your and your baby's best bet.

Acute Health Problems

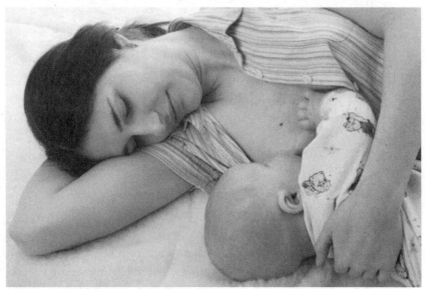

When you're not feeling well, breastfeeding lying down lets you get your rest while protecting your baby from your illness.

FLU OR COLD

When you have a cold or the flu, you may be concerned about infecting your baby. It's important to know that breastfeeding is the only protection your baby has from your illness. Once you have symptoms, your baby has already been exposed because you are most contagious just before your symptoms appear. One of the first things your body does is to produce specific antibodies to fight that illness, some of which go right into your milk. If your baby continues breastfeeding, the antibodies in your milk will either prevent her from catching the illness or, if she does get sick, give her a milder case. If you stop breastfeeding when you start to have symptoms, your baby will be deprived of the only available protection.

Breastfeeding during your illness may also be helpful to you. While you are sick, you can simply tuck your baby into bed with you and not have to worry about getting up to prepare bottles, or worse, going to the store to buy formula. Breastfeeding gives you a way of caring for your baby even when you can do little else.

When you're sick, be sure to drink enough fluids to prevent dehydration, which in severe cases can temporarily affect your milk production. If you are too sick to breastfeed for a few days, see "When You Need to Temporarily Stop Breastfeeding," below, for suggestions.

Chronic Health Problems

Chronic health problems are relatively common. If you have a chronic illness, you may have concerns about breastfeeding. Below we describe several common conditions and offer specific suggestions. But first we have some general advice.

GENERAL SUGGESTIONS FOR MOTHERS WITH CHRONIC ILLNESS

The following guidelines may seem like common sense, but when you're adjusting to caring for an infant while also dealing with a chronic illness, it's good to be reminded to take care of yourself.

Make sure you get enough rest. Fatigue is common for new mothers and even more so for mothers with chronic illnesses. It is essential that you rest regularly. That's where Laws 2, 4, and 5 (about using touch, breastfeeding frequently, and following your own feeding rhythm) will be particularly useful. Nap with your baby. Hold your baby during the day. Learn to nurse lying down so that you can rest during the day. Keep your baby close at night too so that you get more rest and don't need to fully wake up to attend to your baby's needs. And limit the number of guests that you have (especially those you have to entertain).

Accept all offers of help. So often new mothers think that they need to handle everything alone. This is not the time to demonstrate your independence. Being overly fatigued can cause your symptoms to flare. So for the first few weeks or more, accept help.

Get advice about your medications. You might currently be taking one or more prescription medications. Most medications are compatible with breastfeeding, but a few are not. Check with your local La Leche League leader, Australian Breastfeeding Association counselor, or lactation consultant, who generally have access to reference materials that other health care providers do not. Another option is to purchase your own copy of *Medications and Mothers' Milk* (see our Resources section or website for ordering information).

Realize that you may be vulnerable to depression. People with inflammatory disorders, such as lupus, rheumatoid arthritis, and multiple sclerosis (MS), are at higher risk for depression. Be aware that you are probably more vulnerable than most mothers. If you seek support and follow the steps listed above, you have a good chance of preventing an occurrence of depression.

INFLAMMATORY ARTHRITIS, MULTIPLE SCLEROSIS, AND MYASTHENIA GRAVIS

Several kinds of chronic illness are more common for women of childbearing age. These include the various types of inflammatory arthritis (such as lupus, rheumatoid arthritis, or systemic sclerosis) and other illnesses such as MS and myasthenia gravis (MG). These illnesses can cause muscle pain or weakness and painful or swollen joints. But severe fatigue is likely to be your most common challenge, and it's something that people who don't have chronic illnesses sometimes have a hard time understanding. Indeed, having a baby may actually trigger a flare-up of symptoms in the first few months postpartum.

Some may suggest that formula feeding would be easier for you. That decision is yours, of course. But in most cases you might find that it is still better for you to breastfeed. Your baby cannot "catch" your illness through breastfeeding, as these illnesses are caused by a combination of genetics and environmental factors. Indeed, breastfeeding may protect your baby from ever contracting one of them. Below are some suggestions for coping with some of the challenges new mothers with health issues face.

Support your upper-body joints. You will need to find a position that allows you to hold your baby comfortably while not stressing your upper-body joints. Keep a variety of pillows and other supports available so that you don't stress your hands, wrists, elbows, shoulders, or neck. Laid-back breastfeeding can also help.

Watch how you carry your baby. Carrying your baby can also stress your joints and muscles. Front-packs can stress your neck and shoulders. A baby sling is helpful because it takes the stress off your shoulders, wrists, and hands. These are available from many local hospitals or you can find them online (see our website at www.breastfeeding madesimple.com for more information). Cuddling your baby while you are reclining or lying down allows you to connect with her in a way that doesn't stress your joints and muscles and allows you to relax. You might want to ask your physical therapist about some exercises and stretches to counter some of the strain of carrying your baby.

You can care for a baby, even with a chronic illness. Pace yourself, get help and support, and take whatever medications you feel are necessary. (See our website for more information.)

DIABETES

Diabetes is a metabolic disorder caused by your body's inability to make enough insulin or to use the insulin that is available (insulin resistance). If you are diabetic, breastfeeding offers you several important advantages. Generally speaking, diabetes is easier to manage during breastfeeding, as you may require less insulin. And if you had gestational diabetes, breastfeeding can prevent the development of diabetes when you're not pregnant. Even with these advantages, there are some special considerations for the diabetic mother.

Increased risk of hypoglycemia in your baby. About half of all babies born to diabetic mothers have *hypoglycemia*, or low blood sugar. This may require some intervention while you are in the hospital. But frequent breastfeeding may also prevent it.

You may experience a delay in your milk increasing. Some mothers with type 1 diabetes experience a one- to two-day delay in when their milk "comes in." Breastfeeding early and often will help. Even with a delay, you can bring in full milk production.

You may need extra calories. If you have type 1 diabetes, you may need extra calories while you are breastfeeding to help you maintain an adequate milk production. When breastfeeding is established, you may need to adjust how much you eat depending on whether the baby is breastfeeding a little or a lot. You may also need to adjust your dosage of insulin based on how much your baby is breastfeeding. The need to adjust your insulin dose should be obvious as you monitor your blood-sugar levels.

Be alert to possible infections. As a woman with diabetes, you are more prone to all types of infections. (See the "Mastitis" and "Thrush or Yeast Infections" sections in chapter 10.)

Wean gradually. As described in chapter 7, gradual weaning is best for mother and baby. For mothers with diabetes, especially type 1 diabetes, it is also important because of the impact on your blood sugar levels. Gradual weaning will make it easier to keep your diabetes under control.

THYROID DISEASE

The thyroid is a gland that releases a hormone that regulates metabolism. Thyroid levels can be too low or too high. If you are severely fatigued, or find that you can't sit still, a blood test to measure your levels of T3, T4, and TSH can help identify hypo- or hyperthyroidism. If you have thyroid disease, you should be under a doctor's care. If you suspect that you have it, discuss it with your health care provider. Fortunately, in most cases you can continue to breastfeed while being treated.

Symptoms of *hypothyroidism*, or a low level of thyroid hormone, include extreme fatigue, inability to tolerate cold, weight gain, low basal body temperature, dry skin, thinning hair, and depression. You can develop hypothyroidism for the first time in the postpartum period. Low thyroid can also decrease your milk production, but thyroid supplements are compatible with breastfeeding as they simply replace the hormones that your body would normally be producing. And if you take supplements to bring your thyroid to normal levels, you may find that it also increases your milk production.

Hyperthyroidism refers to an overactive thyroid, which results in too-high levels of thyroid hormone in your system. This is a serious medical condition that requires prompt treatment. Most common medications used to treat hyperthyroidism are compatible with breastfeeding. **Note:** Radioactive iodine used for diagnosis or treatment is one of the few medications that breastfeeding mothers should not use. If it is used during a diagnostic test, you must wean for at least forty-eight hours. If it is used as treatment, weaning may need to be permanent. Radioactive materials accumulate in your milk and are passed on to the baby.

Before undergoing treatment for hyperthyroidism, ask your health care provider to first rule out a temporary condition known as *postpartum thyroiditis*. As its name suggests, this condition occurs after childbirth and usually starts with a period of overactive thyroid production, with thyroid levels gradually returning to normal over time.

Unusual Breast or Nipple Anatomy

Every woman is unique. And not surprisingly, there is an amazing diversity of breast sizes and shapes. The overwhelming majority of breasts work just fine. But as with every other organ in the body, sometimes breasts don't function as they should. Some women encounter challenges when they have unusual nipple anatomy or there is not enough milk-producing glandular tissue to allow them to reach full milk production. These situations are described below.

FLAT OR INVERTED NIPPLES

A flat nipple is one that does not protrude or become erect when stimulated or cold. By following Law 3 and using good latch dynamics (see our website at www.breastfeedingmadesimple.com for animation that shows this in motion), flat nipples should not cause breastfeeding problems, especially if at first your baby receives only the breast and is given the chance to learn to breastfeed well for several weeks before receiving bottles or pacifiers.

An inverted nipple is one that when stimulated looks like it is inside out. In most cases of inverted nipples, babies can breastfeed just fine. Again, Law 3 (Better Feel and Flow Happen in the Comfort Zone) and good breastfeeding dynamics are important here. But if a mother has severely inverted nipples, depending on the type and the degree of inversion, breastfeeding may be difficult or impossible. Sometimes mothers have only one flat or inverted nipple, and their babies tend to prefer the other breast.

It's important to remember that babies breastfeed not "nipple feed." If the baby gets a deep latch, taking in a good amount of the areola (the pigmented area around your nipple), flat or inverted nipples will not be a problem in most cases. A *nipple shield* (a flexible silicone nipple with holes in the end worn over the breast during feedings) may be helpful if your baby is having difficulties getting a deep latch. If you are having trouble, contact a lactation specialist for assistance. They have specialized tools, like nipple shields, and know special techniques that can usually help.

INADEQUATE GLANDULAR TISSUE

About one in a thousand women have difficulty establishing full milk production because they do not have enough milk-producing glandular tissue in their breasts. Women who have this condition often have unusually shaped breasts. Your breasts may look tubular (long and slim) rather than rounded, may be very different in size, and your areolas may appear unusual and bulbous. Your breasts may be widely spaced (more than 1.5 inches/3.8 cm apart) and/or did not change size at all when you were pregnant. And you may not have felt any breast fullness after your milk became more plentiful in the first few days postpartum. That being said, you should know that some women who have all these features have been able to establish full milk production. But if your baby is not gaining well, you can try the techniques we suggest to increase your milk production (see chapter 10). If those techniques do not work, you may need to supplement with formula. Even if you cannot bring in full milk production, it's still worth your effort to breastfeed. Remember, some breastfeeding is always better than none.

FIT ISSUES

Sometimes, there is a mismatch between the size of a mother's nipples and the size of her baby's mouth, especially if the mother's nipples are very large and the baby's mouth is very small. In this case, at first it may be difficult or impossible for your baby to latch on deeply to your breast for the first few days or weeks. This can frustrate both mom and baby. If you are experiencing this, take heart. It's a problem that is quickly outgrown, usually during the first month. Once your baby's mouth grows enough, which happens very fast with a newborn, she will be able to latch on deeply and breastfeed. In the meantime, you can establish full milk production with an effective, rental breast pump and feed your baby your milk (see "Pumping to Establish Full Milk Production" later in this chapter for details).

Breast Surgery

Breast surgery is a relatively common procedure in the United States and in other parts of the world. You may have had a biopsy to test for cancer or remove a cyst, or you may have had a breast lift, augmentation, or reduction. And you may be concerned about whether this surgery will keep you from full breastfeeding. The answer is, as with so many other factors, it depends. Here are some general considerations.

LOCATION OF INCISIONS

Where your breast was cut and whether one breast or both were affected can make a tremendous difference in whether you will be able to establish full milk production. Generally speaking, if your surgery involved cutting around the areolas of both breasts, it is more likely to affect breastfeeding as this involves cutting milk ducts and the nerves leading to the nipple. Most critical are the major nerves located at four o'clock and eight o'clock on the areola (known as the *fourth intercostal nerves*).

SURGICAL TECHNIQUE USED

The technique that the surgeon used can also make a difference. If the technique leaves the milk ducts and nerves still attached to the nipple, then your odds of fully breastfeeding are greater. If these are cut, it may be more difficult. If you are reading this before you have surgery, be sure to talk with your surgeon about your desire to breast-feed. Your surgeon may be able to use a technique that minimizes damage to your nerves and ducts.

Learning as much as you can about breastfeeding, no matter what type of surgery you've had, is going to be your best strategy. Some women who, biologically speaking, shouldn't have been able to breast-feed have been able to, because milk ducts can grow back after surgery. The best way for you to know whether you can breastfeed is to give it a try. That being said, it's important for you to know the signs of when your baby is getting enough milk so you'll know if you will need to supplement. Review chapter 4 on how to tell if your baby is getting enough milk. Weigh her frequently, either at your health care provider's office or by renting an accurate electronic baby scale for the first few weeks postpartum. After the initial weight loss from birth to day four, your baby should gain, on average, about 7–8 oz. (200–225 g) a week. Also, keep track of the number of stools, as this is a good indicator of how much milk your baby is getting. If your production is low, review "Low Milk Production" in chapter 10 about how to increase your production.

BREAST AUGMENTATION

Breast augmentation surgery is a relatively common procedure that increases breast size by surgically inserting silicone- or saline-filled implants under the surface of the breast, either above or below the muscles. The incisions can be under the folds in the breasts or near the armpits. These types of incisions are the least likely to have a negative impact on breastfeeding, as they usually leave the milk ducts intact. Incisions around the areola are more likely to interfere with breastfeeding. But even in this situation, some women have established full milk production.

Will silicone harm my baby? Some mothers with silicone implants worry that the implants may leak and silicone will get into their milk. They wonder if formula is a safer choice. If you have this concern, you may be interested to learn that both formula and cow's milk have ten times more silicone than the milk of mothers with implants (Mohrbacher 2010). In addition, silicone itself is considered inert, so even if your baby did ingest some, her digestive tract is unlikely to absorb it. In fact, one form of silicone (simethicone) is given directly to babies as a commonly used colic treatment. So, as usual, you're better off breastfeeding.

BREAST REDUCTION

Breast reduction is another relatively common procedure where fat and tissue are removed from the breast. Unfortunately, this procedure almost always involves cutting at least some of the milk ducts. The more tissue you have removed, the less likely it is that you will be able to establish full milk production. Your chances decrease further if your surgery involved removing the nipple and relocating it to a different place on the breast. However, there is at least one case report of a woman who did bring in full production with both of these factors. This is rare, but not out of the realm of possibility. With time, some severed milk ducts grow back. So the best approach is for you to try breastfeeding while keeping track of how much your baby is getting. Even if you reach partial milk production at most, some breastfeeding is better than none. If you would like to know more about breastfeeding after reduction, we suggest that you get a copy of Diana West's 2001 book *Defining Your Own Success: Breastfeeding After Breast Reduction Surgery* (see our Resource list or website for ordering information or go to her website, www.bfar.org).

Depression, Difficult Birth, Past Sexual Abuse

You may be surprised to learn that your emotional health can have an impact on breastfeeding. In this section, we describe three factors that relate to emotional well-being, and how these can impact your breastfeeding relationship.

DEPRESSION

Depression in the postpartum period is relatively common, affecting 15–25 percent of new mothers worldwide (Kendall-Tackett 2010). The percentages of depressed mothers can be even higher in some high-risk populations. Some of the common symptoms of postpartum depression include sadness, hopelessness, an inability to experience pleasure from everyday activities, excessive emotional sensitivity, sleep and appetite disturbances (too much or too little), agitation, irritability, and an inability to concentrate. It's normal to have some of these symptoms for a day or two. But if they persist for at least two weeks, you might be suffering from depression according to the *Diagnostic and Statistical Manual of Mental Disorders*, 4th ed., text revision (APA 2000).

Depression in new mothers can be caused by a whole range of factors. These can be broken down into roughly five categories:

- physiological factors, such as stress, pain, fatigue, and inflammation

- negative birth experiences (see, for example, "Difficult Birth," below)

- infant characteristics, such as temperament, prematurity, and disability

- psychological factors, such as self-esteem and previous episodes of depression

- social factors, such as childhood loss and abuse, lack of support, and low income (Kendall-Tackett 2010)

Much more information is available on our website (www.breast feedingmadesimple.com). If you are depressed, there are a few things that are important for you to keep in mind.

Breastfeeding lowers your risk of depression. In a recent review of 49 studies, researchers Dennis and McQueen (2009) found that formula-feeding mothers had higher rates of depression than their breastfeeding counterparts. Because it lowers stress, breastfeeding protects you. But having breastfeeding *problems* increases your risk, so it's important for those to be addressed promptly.

Depression can influence how you relate to your baby. Although depression can influence your relationship with your baby, breastfeeding protects your baby while you are depressed. Dozens of studies have documented that depression can have a negative impact on how you respond to your baby. Depressed mothers are often not as tuned in to their babies' cues or as positive when interacting with their babies, and tend to make eye contact less often. However, one study found that breastfeeding helped protect babies from the negative effects of their mothers' depression (Jones, McFall, and Diego 2004). It's much more difficult to be emotionally disconnected from a breastfeeding baby. This is one more important reason to continue breastfeeding.

Breastfeeding helps you interact more positively. Of all the laws we've described, Law 2, which encourages touch (see chapter 2) is going to be the most helpful for you. If skin to skin is too intense, holding your baby while you are clothed can be helpful. Mothers who carry their babies by wearing them become more positive with them and more responsive to their cues. Also, having your baby near when you sleep is going to be helpful since you will be able to respond without being fully awake. Some will tell you that you need to wean, at least at night, so you can get more sleep. You may be surprised to learn that when the sleep of breastfeeding, formula-feeding, and mixed-feeding mothers were studied, the exclusively breastfeeding mothers got more sleep (Doan et al. 2007). And in a recent article on post-partum depression, sleep disturbance, and infant sleep, researchers indicated that exclusive breastfeeding protected the mothers from depression (Dorheim et al. 2009). So the bottom line is that weaning at night (which may be recommended by friends and family) may, in fact, prolong your depression.

Your friends and family may urge you to quit breastfeeding. Despite the point just mentioned, many in your life may "give you permission" to stop breastfeeding, even if you want to continue. That can be devastating advice. Actress Brooke Shields, in her book *Down Came the Rain*, described her experience of postpartum depression, putting it this way:

> If I were to eliminate [breastfeeding], I might have no hope of coming through this nightmare. I was hanging on to breastfeeding as my lifeline (quoted in McCarter-Spaulding and Horowitz 2007, 80).

Get support. This is another time when you don't want to go it alone. It's important that you seek support from your partner, family, or friends. But, tying into the point above, you might need to gently let your friends and family know that telling you to wean is not helping. When support works well, it can lessen your depression and also help you be more positive with your baby. Try to find a local mothers' group or mother-to-mother breastfeeding group. Some moms have found that the women they meet in their childbirth education class can be a great source of support. And don't rule out online support. This is especially important where local in-person support is not available.

Most treatments for depression are compatible with breastfeeding. Getting help for your depression is going to benefit both you and your baby. Of the medications that are compatible with breastfeeding, Zoloft (sertraline), Paxil (paroxetine), and Lexapro (escitalopram) have the best safety records for breastfeeding, with less than one percent of your dosage reaching your baby. But even Prozac (fluoxetine), which initially raised some concern, now has more than twenty years' worth of data indicating that it is not harmful to breastfeeding babies (Hale 2010; Kendall-Tackett and Hale 2010). There are also a number of nondrug treatments that are effective for even major depression, including omega-3 supplementation, exercise, psychotherapy, bright light, social support, and Saint-John's-wort (Kendall-Tackett 2008, 2010, forthcoming). If you decide on a nondrug option, you should discuss it with your health care provider.

See our website (www.breastfeedingmadesimple.com) for a short video clip about postpartum depression and for handouts and a full listing of your medications and nondrug treatment options. The impact of each of these treatments on breastfeeding is also described. Postpartum Support International (www.postpartum.net) also keeps a listing of counselors who specialize in perinatal mental health. This is a great resource. But as is true with any health care provider, these counselors may or may not be knowledgeable about breastfeeding or supportive of your desire to continue. It's good to be aware of your options before you seek care.

In closing, if you are depressed, we want you to know three final things:

1. You are not alone.

2. There is help available.

3. If you want to continue breastfeeding, you can and should.

DIFFICULT BIRTH

A difficult birth can be physically and emotionally challenging. Sometimes the experiences are sufficiently frightening or life-threatening to cause depression or post-traumatic stress disorder (PTSD). On top of all that, women may also develop breastfeeding problems. If breastfeeding is not going well, don't wait before you get some help. We've worked with enough women to tell you confidently that most of these problems are solvable, even if you've had a really difficult beginning.

There are three breastfeeding problems that seem to be more common following a difficult birth: delayed onset of lactation, temporary low milk production, and breast refusal. All of these problems are discussed in more detail in chapter 10, so we'll mention them only briefly here.

Delayed onset of lactation. A highly stressful birth can delay when your milk increases. A study in Guatemala found that women who had high levels of the stress hormone cortisol after a difficult birth had a delay of several days (Grajeda and Perez-Escamilla 2002). Cesarean births can also delay when you first breastfeed. Although breastfeeding before the epidural wears off is most comfortable, not all mothers have this opportunity. Some mothers are not given their babies for several hours, or even overnight, after delivery. But the good news is that in at least one study, this delay did not seem to have any long-term effects on mothers' ability to breastfeed or how long they breastfed (Rowe-Murray and Fisher 2002).

Low milk production. Researchers are starting to realize that the physiological aspects of a difficult birth can have an impact on breastfeeding. For example, severe postpartum hemorrhage can sometimes delay milk production. Low milk production might occur if you were under severe stress during your labor and delivery or had a mild to moderate postpartum hemorrhage (Willis and Livingstone 1995).

Breast refusal. Breastfeeding success is often even more important to mothers after a difficult birth than when birth goes smoothly. But related issues, such as separation of mother and baby and early supplementation, may cause difficulties for you postpartum. Sometimes a baby will respond to a traumatic birth by actively refusing her mother's breasts. If your baby is refusing to breastfeed, you may conclude that your baby does not like you, which can be devastating.

What to do if you are having problems. Fortunately, all of these problems are solvable. But there are a few things that you must do:

- *Protect your milk production.* If your baby is not breastfeeding well or is refusing the breast, you must protect your production. That may mean renting a pump until things get back on track. Plan to remove milk from your breasts eight to twelve times a day to bring in a good production. Law 4, *More breastfeeding at first means more milk later,* is going to be helpful here, with a pump substituting for your baby.

- *Feed the baby.* If your milk production is significantly lower than it should be, you may need to supplement with formula for a few days. While this is not ideal, it may be necessary. Keep your long-term goals in mind.

- *Have lots of contact with your baby.* As outlined by Laws 1 and 2, using your baby's hardwiring and using touch are going to be especially relevant in your situation. Hold your baby and have lots of skin-to-skin contact, unless that feels too overwhelming. Allow your baby to practice breastfeeding when she is not particularly hungry but is in a quiet, alert state, or even when she is drowsy or in a light sleep. Babies who are calm and not frantically hungry can, in most cases, be coaxed onto the breast, especially in laid-back positions that trigger their inborn feeding reflexes. Make the breast a pleasant place to be.

- *Rule out physical trauma to the baby.* Sometimes after a difficult delivery, babies may be suffering from a birth-related injury. They may be sore from a vacuum extraction or forceps delivery. They may have a neck injury, torticollis (a pulled neck muscle caused by a confined position in the womb), broken collarbone (clavicle), or another physical issue. Being held in a certain way for breastfeeding may be painful. Watch your baby and see if that appears to be so. No one eats well when in pain, and you can make some adjustments accordingly.

- *Recognize the meaning of your baby's behavior.* If your baby is refusing the breast or not breastfeeding well, it doesn't mean she does not like breastfeeding—or you. While it is natural for mothers to sometimes feel that way, make the rational adult part of your brain keep repeating that it's simply not true. The more contact that you can have with your baby during this time, the better. Soon you will realize that your baby not only likes you but actually prefers you to all other people.

If you are interested in more information, we refer you to an article on our website (www.breastfeedingmadesimple.com), "Making Peace with Your Birth Experience."

PAST SEXUAL ABUSE OR SEXUAL ASSAULT

For adult survivors of sexual abuse or assault, breastfeeding can also pose challenges. Unfortunately, sexual abuse and assault are relatively common experiences, affecting approximately 20–25 percent of women (Kendall-Tackett 2010; Kendall-Tackett 2004). The reactions of abuse survivors to breastfeeding run the whole range of responses, from really disliking breastfeeding to finding it tremendously healing.

Some people assume that survivors of sexual trauma do not want to breastfeed. But that is not what researchers have found. Two studies have found that pregnant abuse survivors were more likely to say that they planned to breastfeed (Benedict, Paine, and Paine 1994) and were more likely to start breastfeeding in the hospital (Prentice et al. 2002) compared with nonabused women. In a more recent study, the same percentage of sexual trauma survivors were breastfeeding as were women with no history of trauma (Kendall-Tackett and Hale 2010, in press).

If you are an abuse survivor who wants to breastfeed, we'd like to congratulate you for making a positive life choice to overcome your past and to parent well. But we also want to acknowledge that you may face some unique challenges.

We've included both sexual abuse and assault in this section because we have found that both can make a difference. Sexual abuse is often something that happens within the family and can include everything from fondling to rape. Sexual assault is often outside the family and can also include attacks by peers. We have found that women have similar reactions to both of these experiences.

If you are having a hard time with breastfeeding, we have some specific suggestions. But mostly we suggest that you give yourself permission to do whatever works for and helps you. If you are having difficulties, your first step is to try to figure out what makes you uncomfortable. Is it nighttime feeding? Is it your baby touching other parts of your body while nursing? Is it latching on? Or all of the above? The intense physical contact of breastfeeding may be very uncomfortable for trauma survivors in general. You might find breastfeeding painful because your abuse experience lowered your pain threshold. The act of breastfeeding may also trigger flashbacks. There is a whole range of things that might be uncomfortable for you. If you're not sure, try keeping a diary for a week or so to see if you can identify some specific triggers.

Can you address the problem? If skin-to-skin contact is bothering you, can you put a towel or cloth between you and the baby? Can you avoid the feedings that make you uncomfortable? Nighttime feedings are often a good candidate. Would you be more comfortable if you pumped and fed your baby with a bottle? Can you hold baby's other hand while breastfeeding to keep her from touching your body? Can you distract yourself with TV or a book while breastfeeding (many mothers have told us that this works well for them)? Experiment and find out what helps.

Remember that some breastfeeding is better than none. You may not be able to fully breastfeed, but every little bit helps, even if you must pump milk and use a bottle, even if you are only breastfeeding once a day. Some abuse survivors find that they never love breastfeeding but they learn to tolerate it. And that may be a more realistic goal for you.

Past abuse does not have to influence the rest of your life. We have both known many abuse survivors who have gone on to become wonderful mothers. We're confident that you can, too.

We have many resources on our website (www.breastfeedingmade-simple.com) for abuse survivors. We would also like to recommend the books *Survivor Moms*, by Mickey Sperlich and Julia Seng, and *When Abuse Survivors Give Birth*, by Penny Simkin and Phyllis Klaus (see our Resources section for details).

Special Situations: Baby

Babies may also have some physical challenges that influence their ability to breastfeed. These can be temporary, such as colds or the flu, or longer term, such as prematurity, Down syndrome, cleft palate, or tongue-tie. In this section, we also describe what to do when you need to temporarily stop breastfeeding and how to bring in full milk production with a pump.

Acute or Chronic Health Problems

Sometimes even breastfed babies become sick. Or your baby may have a chronic health problem. In either case, as we explained in the introduction, the health outcomes of breastfeeding are better for you and your baby than using nonhuman milks. However, there may be some challenges, so here are suggestions on how to cope.

COLDS, FLU, EAR INFECTION

When your baby has a cold or the flu, she may not want to breastfeed. Breastfeeding may be difficult when she has a stuffy nose because she can't breathe when she closes her mouth over your breast. Ear infections can also make her uncomfortable, especially when she is lying on her side. And the suction she creates to breastfeed can make her ears hurt. Even if she's uncomfortable, your milk is still the easiest food for her to handle, will better prevent dehydration, and will help her recover more quickly. Here are some strategies:

- Breastfeed your baby in a different position. Sometimes laid-back positions or sitting up are more comfortable for babies with lots of congestion. Keep your baby upright at other times as well for better drainage of nasal passages.

- Breastfeed in a room with high humidity, either from a vaporizer or a running shower.

- Short, frequent feedings may be easier for your baby to manage.

- If your baby is very congested, contact her health care provider for other suggestions.

If your baby is refusing to nurse, you need to express your milk and give it to her another way. Be sure to drain your breasts, as often as you would have breastfed, to keep up your milk production and prevent mastitis. (See "When You Need to Temporarily Stop Breastfeeding" below.)

DIARRHEA, VOMITING, REFLUX DISEASE

Although it is less likely, breastfed babies sometimes develop these health problems. Breastfeeding is still your best approach.

Diarrhea. Diarrhea can develop from a variety of causes. Before assuming this is your baby's problem, first be sure that it is actual diarrhea and not simply the normal loose stools of a breastfed baby. It's real diarrhea if your baby has twelve to sixteen stools in a day, if the stools are watery with no substance, or if the stools suddenly seem a lot stinkier (normal stools of a breastfed baby have a mild scent). If your baby has green, frothy stools, refer to the section "Overabundant Milk Production" in chapter 10 for strategies.

Continuing to breastfeed is the best thing you can do if your baby has diarrhea. This is true in all but some highly unusual situations (such as *galactosemia*, a rare metabolic disorder). In fact, although doctors used to tell mothers to wean temporarily when their babies had diarrhea, researchers have discovered that that advice is not helpful.

Note: You should be alert to signs of dehydration in a newborn, such as a weak cry, fewer than two wet diapers in a day, a sunken or depressed-looking *fontanel* (the soft spot on the head), dry eyes or mouth, and skin that stays pinched-looking after you gently pinch it. If you see these signs, contact your baby's doctor immediately.

Vomiting. Even healthy babies can spit up a lot of milk. If your baby is showing no other signs of illness, has at least three to four bowel movements a day (the size of a U.S. quarter [2.5 cm] or larger), and is gaining weight well, this is no cause for concern. During the first four months, breastfed babies average a weight gain of about 7–8 oz. (200–225 g) a week. (This weight gain slows down as they get older.) If your baby is not gaining well, or if you are just concerned, contact your baby's health care provider. You might also try experimenting with smaller, more frequent breastfeedings to see if that cuts down on the amount of spit-up. Sometimes babies spit up because of mothers' desire to "top off" their babies, or make them really full. This can also happen when a fast feeder is cajoled into breastfeeding longer, until the "right" number of minutes has passed. This extra milk has to go somewhere—in this case, back out.

If your baby is vomiting a lot because she is sick, you might try expressing some milk and letting your baby nurse on an almost-drained breast for comfort. That way, your baby will still get some milk and will have the comfort of breastfeeding. She may be able to tolerate smaller, frequent feedings better than the larger feedings that she is used to.

You do not have to wean or suspend breastfeeding when your baby is vomiting. This used to be the standard advice, but now research has demonstrated that this is not beneficial (Mohrbacher 2010). Unlike nonhuman milks, your milk is quickly and easily absorbed by your baby. You will want to watch for signs of dehydration (see above). If you see any, be sure to contact your baby's health care provider immediately.

Reflux disease. *Gastroesophageal reflux disease* (GERD) is another health issue that can develop in the first year of life. Reflux occurs when stomach acid backs up into the esophagus, which is normal in all children and adults. However, when it damages these delicate tissues, it is considered a disease. Your baby may choke or cough while eating. Or she may arch back, turn her head, or flatten out, rather than cuddle and settle in when you try to feed her. She may have intense periods of crying during and after feedings. And finally, she may refuse to feed at all. All of these behaviors can be distressing to both you and your baby, but they are no reflection on you or your mothering skills. She is most likely in pain.

If you and your baby's health care provider suspect reflux, you may decide on a trial of medication. If it helps, this can confirm reflux. There are also other strategies that can be helpful. Take advantage of gravity to keep your baby's stomach acid where it should be—in the stomach. To do this, always keep your baby's head higher than her bottom, and avoid bending your baby in the middle, such as when she is in a car seat, since this can also push on the stomach, making the acid rise.

A baby sling or carrier can be helpful to keep your baby upright. Use breastfeeding holds that keep your baby's head higher than her bottom. You may want to put a firm wedge under your baby to elevate her head while she sleeps. **Note:** Never use a pillow under your baby as it's unsafe.

Sometimes mothers find that their babies sleep better in their bouncers. You might also find it helpful to elevate your baby's changing surface so her head is higher, and turn your baby side to side rather than bending her in the middle when changing diapers. Also, shorter, more frequent feedings may help your baby because her stomach won't be as full.

Two strategies that don't seem to work for babies with reflux are adding thickeners to their feedings and/or putting them on formula. Thickeners are unhelpful because they are introducing something other than human milk into the baby's immature gut. This can cause more problems than it solves. Also, if thickeners are mixed with human milk, the active enzymes in human milk break them down quickly. Similarly, using formula simply compounds your baby's problems since you are adding foreign proteins, which are harder to handle, to your baby's system. Research indicates that babies with reflux do better on human milk than on formula because human milk passes through the stomach faster, resulting in fewer symptoms (Mohrbacher 2010).

Prematurity, Down Syndrome, Cleft Lip or Palate, Tongue-Tie

Another challenging situation some mothers face is having a baby who is physically compromised. Fortunately, nearly all of these babies can eventually breastfeed. And right from the start, your milk can make a difference in how healthy your baby is and when she can come home from the hospital.

PREMATURITY

Having a premature or low-birth-weight baby can be a very frightening experience. Premature babies can be low birth weight (3.3–5 lbs.; 1,500–2,500 g), very low birth weight (less than 3.3 lbs.; 1,500 g), or extremely low birth weight (less than 2.3 lbs.; 1,000 g). You may be in shock after you've had your baby. Mothers often report feeling frightened, angry, guilty, and helpless. In one study, 44 percent of mothers had symptoms of acute stress disorder, the precursor syndrome to PTSD (Shaw et al. 2006). You may feel completely overwhelmed by the hospital environment and the emergency nature of your baby's birth. These feelings are normal. However, there are also some very important things that you can do to help your baby.

Your milk works like a medicine for your baby. Your body will produce exactly what your baby needs, starting with colostrum. As the mother of a premature baby, your milk is higher in anti-infective properties, nitrogen, protein nitrogen, sodium, chloride, iron, and fatty acids than mothers of full-term babies (Mohrbacher 2010). It also has even higher concentrations of those nonfood aspects of your milk that promote normal immune and digestive function than the milk of mothers of full-term babies. Your milk is just what your baby needs to grow and thrive. Research has found that preemies fed nonhuman milks have more life-threatening infections and lower intelligence as they mature (Mohrbacher 2010).

Protect your milk production. Since premature babies can have difficulty breastfeeding, you will need to begin pumping immediately. Little babies sometimes tire easily and doze off before they have had enough to eat. Some cannot be brought to breast at all in the early weeks. Even if this is the case, your baby can be fed with your milk. See "Pumping to Establish Full Milk Production" later in this chapter for instructions.

Spend as much time as you can skin to skin with your baby. Fortunately, there have been some positive changes in the way that hospitals handle premature babies. In the bad old days, mothers were kept away from their babies until it was close to time for them to go home. Is it any wonder that mothers often felt disconnected from their babies and that it was necessary for "experts" to care for them?

In chapter 2, we described how skin-to-skin contact can help your baby grow and thrive. This simple technique increased the survival rate of premature babies in developing countries such as Colombia and South Africa. And it has been helpful in industrialized countries, as well. Babies who were held skin to skin gained weight faster, had less stress, and went home sooner. These babies also were able to breastfeed sooner. A review of more than thirty studies concluded that preterm babies who spend more time in skin-to-skin contact after birth are more likely to breastfeed and to breastfeed longer (Moore, Anderson, and Bergman 2007). Skin-to-skin contact has also been found to increase milk production in mothers who are pumping for their preterm babies (Hurst et al. 1997).

Skin-to-skin contact also increased mothers' feelings of confidence, decreased their sense of helplessness and depression, and helped them connect with their babies. Since you are protecting your milk production by pumping, you can relax and enjoy your baby's initial attempts at breastfeeding, even if she isn't yet capable of fully feeding at the breast in the early days or weeks. Spending lots of time holding your baby can give you many opportunities to practice throughout the day. Research has found practice at the breast to be the most important factor in how quickly a premature baby can begin fully breastfeeding (Cunha et al. 2009). In Sweden, where mothers are encouraged to give their preemies lots of practice time at the breast from as young as twenty-nine weeks gestation, 85 percent of the hospitalized premature babies exclusively breastfeed (Nyqvist 2008). Review chapter 2 for more information, and check out the resources on our website (www.breastfeedingmadesimple.com).

Get support. Having a premature baby can be a difficult experience. Several recent studies have found that parents who have peer support feel less depressed and more confident as mothers (Kendall-Tackett 2010). Find out what sources of support are available locally or online. Reaching out to others can make a big difference in how well you cope and the ease of your transition into motherhood.

DOWN SYNDROME

Mothers of babies with Down syndrome can also suffer from shock and denial in the hours after their babies' births—especially if they didn't know before the baby was born. Babies with Down syndrome may also have some health issues, such as heart problems, that require immediate intervention. If so, they may need to be transferred to another hospital and be separated from you. This can be highly stressful for mothers who experience it. Fortunately, there are some steps that you can take to help you breastfeed your baby.

Your milk protects your baby. Since babies with Down syndrome are prone to respiratory infections and bowel problems, breastfeeding can help maintain good health. Even if you must pump in the beginning, your milk offers important protection.

Breastfeeding helps mouth and tongue coordination. Feeding your baby at the breast can help her gain better tongue control and can contribute to a more normal development of her facial muscles.

Touch will help you and your baby. You might be concerned about how you will mother your baby. Skin-to-skin contact, or holding your baby while you are lightly clothed, is a great place to start. It will increase your milk production and help you tune in to your baby's cues. (Review chapter 2 for more specific suggestions on skin-to-skin contact.)

Offer your breast many times a day. Since babies with Down syndrome can be sleepy at the breast, you may find that your baby does better when she has short, frequent feedings throughout the day. If your baby is not gaining weight well, you can pump the higher-fat milk available at the end of the pumping into a separate container and provide it for your baby in a bottle, at-breast supplementer (see below), or other feeding device to give her extra calories.

Since babies with Down syndrome often have problems with tongue thrusting, it may be more challenging to get your baby latched on deeply. It may take a few extra tries, so you will want to start trying to latch your baby on before she is very hungry. Squeeze a few drops of milk onto your breast and encourage your baby to open wide.

Babies with Down syndrome also tend to have low muscle tone in their facial muscles. Because of this, they may need extra support when they are at the breast. Slide your fingers under your breast, forming a U. Slide your fingers forward so that your thumb and index finger are each on your baby's cheek (one on each side) to give her the extra support she needs to stay on the breast. Support your baby's chin at the bottom of the U. This is called the *Dancer hand position* (see the illustration on the next page).

If your baby is choking while breastfeeding, use a laid-back breastfeeding position (see chapter 3) so that gravity will help slow milk flow. You can do this in a chair, leaning back, or you can support yourself with pillows in bed. Your baby may swallow a lot of air when she nurses so may need to be burped more often than a baby without Down syndrome.

Breastfeeding is most definitely possible and desirable for the baby with Down syndrome. As your baby increases in muscle tone, breastfeeding will become easier and you'll be able to relax and enjoy the special closeness of the breastfeeding relationship.

CLEFT LIP OR PALATE

A *cleft* is an opening, and a cleft lip or palate refers to an opening in the lip or palate. These conditions can occur separately or together. If a baby has a cleft lip alone, this usually presents a more minor challenge to breastfeeding. Often all a mother needs to do is to use her thumb to plug the opening in the lip to maintain suction during breastfeedings. Cleft lips are usually surgically corrected at a young age, sometimes even right after birth.

But there are more serious feeding issues for a baby with a cleft palate. Until the opening is repaired, it can be challenging for your baby to feed either at the breast or with a bottle, because she cannot create suction in her mouth to keep the breast or bottle in place or draw out the milk. However, with patience and practice, at least partial breastfeeding is possible, and it is well worth the effort.

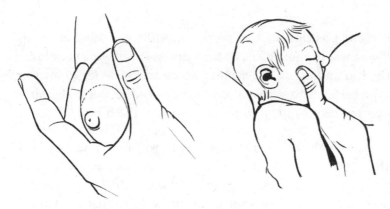

The Dancer hand position can be used to help special needs babies breast-feed. (©2010 Anna Mohrbacher, used with permission)

Your milk protects your baby. Because the cleft allows liquid to flow into their ear canals, babies with cleft palates are more prone to ear infections than babies without a cleft. Even partial human milk feedings can limit the number of infections your baby has and make her healthier overall. In addition, if your milk leaks into your baby's nose (which is a common problem for babies with a cleft palate), it will be much less irritating to these delicate tissues than formula.

Even if babies cannot fully feed at the breast, the act of breastfeeding helps strengthen and develop their facial muscles. Feeding at the breast is also comforting in a way that bottlefeeding is not (and babies with clefts often cannot use pacifiers).

In the lactation field, we used to be a lot more optimistic about whether babies with cleft palates could fully breastfeed. More recent research has indicated that full breastfeeding may be an elusive goal for all but a few. But partial breastfeeding and exclusive human milk feeding is entirely possible—especially if you work toward that goal from the beginning. Here are some things to try.

Pump to establish full milk production. Babies with a cleft palate are not able to drain the breast effectively, so consider the pump to be your primary way of establishing full milk production and think of breastfeeding as an "extra." Give the pumped milk to your baby using another feeding method (see "Alternatives to Feeding at the Breast," below).

Try different positions. Experiment with different positions at the breast. Some will be more effective than others in allowing your breast to fill the gap and create the suction necessary to better drain your breast. For babies with a cleft lip, you may need to put a thumb or finger over the baby's top lip to create suction at the breast.

Support your baby's jaw. One technique you may find helpful is called the "Dancer hand position" (illustrated on previous page). Slide your fingers under your breast, forming a U. Your baby's chin should be at the bottom of the U. Slide your fingers forward so that your thumb and index finger are each on your baby's cheeks (one on each side) to give her the extra support she needs to stay on the breast.

Use adaptive equipment. Some mothers have found it helpful to have a *palatal obturator* made for their baby. This is a special mouth appliance that can help babies feed more normally by providing a firm surface at the roof of the mouth. A *Haberman feeder* can also be helpful. This is a bottle designed for babies with feeding difficulties. The baby controls the milk flow with compression rather than suction, and it can be adjusted for a slower or faster flow.

Realize that feeding will take time. Whether feeding at the breast or with a bottle, feedings typically take two to three times longer for a baby with a cleft palate, so you should plan accordingly.

Breastfeed before and after surgery. At some point, your baby will have surgery to repair the cleft. Find out what your surgeon's guidelines are in terms of feeding before or after surgery. Most hospitals today allow breastfeeding up to four hours before surgery and as soon as a baby wakes from anesthesia. Refer your surgeon to the book *Breastfeeding: A Guide for the Medical Profession* (Lawrence and Lawrence 2005) if they have questions.

TONGUE-TIE

If your baby has trouble breastfeeding, it may be because she has an abnormally short *frenulum* or a "tongue-tie." The frenulum is that stringy membrane under your baby's tongue. If that is tight, it can prevent your baby's tongue from cupping under the breast and also from extending over your baby's lower gum during feedings (you can have a helper check for this while you're breastfeeding). There are also other types of tongue-tie that restrict the movement of the back or middle of the tongue, reducing baby's breastfeeding effectiveness. Possible indicators of this include the following:

- nipple pain or trauma despite a deep latch

- clicking sounds and/or difficulty staying on the breast

- slow weight gain

If you suspect that this may be an issue for your baby, take a look at her tongue when her mouth is open. Babies with tongue-tie often have tongues that dip in the middle, forming a heart shape. Or it may be impossible for your baby to raise her tongue to the roof of her mouth.

The treatment for tongue-tie is to clip the frenulum, the membrane under the tongue. That sounds much worse than it is for your baby. There are few nerves and blood vessels in that part of the body, and the procedure is usually done quickly in a doctor's office with little or no need for anesthesia. Your baby should be able to nurse immediately after the procedure. What you will notice is an amazing decrease in pain while your baby is at the breast. Oral surgeons, some dentists, pediatricians, or ear, nose, and throat specialists can perform this procedure. Ask the breastfeeding specialists in your community. For more information, see the article on our website, www.breastfeedingmade-simple.com, on tongue-tie (Coryllos, Genna, and Salloum, 2004). It has pictures and a good explanation of the procedure. Print this information out and discuss it with your baby's doctor.

When You Need to Temporarily Stop Breastfeeding

If you need to temporarily stop breastfeeding because you or your baby are sick, or because you need to take a medication that is incompatible with breastfeeding, there are some steps that you can take to help both you and your baby:

- *Express your milk as many times per day as you would breastfeed.* Your body is used to making milk in certain amounts. In order to maintain your production, you will need to drain your breasts about as often as you would have while breastfeeding. If you don't do this, you are at increased risk of engorgement and mastitis. Don't wait until your breasts feel full to start expressing your milk. Full breasts are a signal to your body to slow production (see chapter 6).

- *Use a good-quality pump with double-pumping attachments*, which allow you to pump both breasts at once. The best way to maintain your production is with a rental pump or a single-user pump that provides at least forty to sixty suction-and-release cycles per minute. Other methods of breast draining may not be adequate for maintaining your production unless you are already very skilled at them.

- *Breastfeed long and often once you start again.* If you find that you're not able to fit in enough pumpings, you might find that your production is down. Once your baby is at the breast again, bring your production back up with long, frequent breastfeedings. Use skin-to-skin contact and frequent feedings to reestablish your production (see laws 2 and 4). If low production continues to be a problem, you might need to use an herb or medication to increase your production (see "Low Milk Production" in chapter 10). If your baby is refusing to breastfeed, see "Breast Refusal or Nursing Strike" in chapter 10 for suggestions.

Alternatives to Feeding at the Breast

Even mothers who are breastfeeding sometimes need a way to feed their babies other than at the breast. Perhaps your baby is in the hospital and either tires quickly at the breast or is too small to breastfeed. Perhaps you need to return to work, and your care provider needs to feed your baby. Perhaps you need to supplement your baby until your milk production increases. Or maybe you are an adoptive mother and need to supplement as you build your own milk production. Whatever the situation, you have a variety of options, including, of course, bottles. (See chapter 9 for more information on using bottles.)

If you're working with a lactation consultant, he or she may have some strong opinions about how feedings should be supplemented. Having worked with lots of mothers, we can tell you that there are many shades of gray when it comes to selecting a feeding method. What works well for one family is less effective for another. We encourage you to be flexible and see what works well for you.

Bottle

Although you may automatically think of a bottle, there are actually many ways to supplement a baby. If a baby is one month old or older and has been breastfeeding well, depending on circumstance, a bottle may be your best choice. If your baby is younger than a month and is not breastfeeding well, you might consider other options.

Spoon, Cup, Eyedropper, or Feeding Syringe

The simplest is an ordinary spoon. Your baby can lick or sip your milk or colostrum from the spoon. You can also use a small cup: one that you own (such as those that come on the top of children's liquid medications) or one that you buy that is specially designed to feed a baby. You can also use an eyedropper or feeding syringe. These allow you to slowly drip your breast milk or supplemental formula into your baby's mouth.

With each of these options, there are a few things to keep in mind:

- Wait until your baby is alert and awake before trying to feed her. Your baby needs to be awake enough to drink the milk you offer.

- Swaddle or wrap your baby to keep her from bumping your feeding device. Since it is much easier to spill, you will want to make sure that your baby's hands are not free.

- Hold your baby upright while feeding. Sitting up makes it easier for your baby to take the milk.

- Don't pour the milk into your baby's mouth. Allow her to lick or sip it. That way, your baby can set the pace and not feel overwhelmed by the feeding. Don't offer more until your baby has had a chance to swallow.

The techniques we've described here are often most appropriate for newborns. Once your baby gets to be a few weeks or months old, you may find that your baby is less receptive to these approaches.

At-Breast Supplementer

Another option is an *at-breast supplementer*. This is a device that includes a bottle or pouch that, in some models, you wear around your neck and in others, sits on a surface next to you. The bottle is filled with your milk or formula, and there is thin tubing that leads from the container to your breast. When your baby latches on to your breast, she also takes the tubing. The supplement flows through the tubing while she is breastfeeding.

At-breast supplementers may be used in a variety of situations, such as when your baby is premature or has a cleft palate. Your baby may be ill and have a weak suck, meaning she does not drain your breasts well enough for you to make enough milk. Your production may be low after cutting back on breastfeeding or weaning. Or you may use one of these supplementers if you are nursing an adopted baby. While a supplementer can be a great solution for some mothers, others don't like it. Keep in mind that this is only one of your possible options. Talk with your local lactation consultant or your local hospital if you'd like to give this a try.

Pumping to Establish Full Milk Production

If for some reason your baby cannot breastfeed or is ineffective at the breast, you can stimulate full milk production with a pump. Here are some suggestions to help you:

- *Start by pumping with a rental pump at least eight to ten times every twenty-four hours.* This is as many times per day as your baby would be nursing. Use a double-pumping kit to pump both breasts at once. Some suggest mothers put eight or ten candies or other treats next to their pump each day as a visual reminder to make sure to fit in enough pumpings.

- *Pump both breasts at least ten to fifteen minutes per pumping session.* Do this for the first few days after birth until your milk increases. After that, as many times per day as you can fit it in, pump both breasts for two minutes after you see the last drop of milk, or up to thirty minutes total. Draining the breasts more fully increases your milk production faster (see chapter 6). Manually expressing milk after pumping can also help. Do this until you have full milk production, ideally by days ten to fourteen. At that time, you can go back to pumping both breasts ten to fifteen minutes.

- *Focus on the number of pumpings per day, not the time between pumpings.* If you think in terms of the intervals between pumpings (for instance, every two or three hours), it is too easy for the number of pumpings to drop without your realizing it. Instead, when planning your day, think: "How can I fit in my ten or so pumpings?" If you can't pump during part of the day, pump every hour when you can to meet your goal.

- *Most women can cut back on the number of pumpings once they establish full production.* The maximum amount of human milk a baby typically takes per day is 25–35 oz. (750–1,050 ml). Your goal should be to pump this much milk by ten to fourteen days after birth, no matter how much your baby is taking. It takes much more work to increase to a full production if you wait longer than this. Once you're pumping at least 25–35 oz. (750–1,050 ml) a day, try cutting back to five to seven pumping sessions a day. Most women can maintain their production at this level of pumping for as long as they choose. If your production starts to decrease, this means you probably have a small breast storage capacity (see chapter 6) and you'll need to increase the number of pumpings to increase and maintain your production.

- *Once you have full production, you may not need to pump during your normal sleeping hours.* Until you have full production, pump at least once during the night and don't go longer than five hours between pumping sessions. Once you have full production, if your breast storage capacity is large enough, you may be able to pump right before bed and first thing in the morning without your milk production dropping. If you can do this without discomfort, go ahead.

How to Wean from Pumping

If your baby is not breastfeeding and you are ready to wean from pumping, you can do it painlessly and safely using the same principles we described in chapter 7. Gradually cut back on pumping sessions by eliminating one daily pumping, give your body two to three days to adjust, and then eliminate another daily pumping. Repeat until you have eliminated all your pumping sessions, leaving the one before bedtime and the one when you get up for last. Another weaning strategy is to stop pumping before you get as much milk as usual. For example, if you normally get 3 oz. (90 ml) at a pumping, stop at 2 oz. (60 ml) at each session. With either of these approaches (or a combination of both), if you feel full at any time, pump to comfort—not a full pumping, but long enough so that your breasts feel more comfortable. Leaving your breasts feeling too full can cause pain and mastitis (see chapter 7). If your weaning is gradual enough, it should always be comfortable.

Epilogue: You're on Your Way

Having a baby is one of life's major transitions and learning to breast-feed can take patience and persistence, especially if you haven't had the chance to learn it by watching mothers breastfeed during your growing-up years. If your learning is just now beginning, you may need to review the information we shared with you many times as you get the hang of breastfeeding. We hope you find it helpful.

Also be sure to check out our website, www.breastfeedingmade simple.com, which contains lots of information that just wouldn't fit in this book. It includes details about special circumstances, video clips, handouts, and much, much more.

You're most definitely on your way! Give your sweet baby a kiss for us. Your baby is very lucky you are learning what you need to know to make breastfeeding work. Many mothers think about the health effects of breastfeeding to stay motivated as they work their way through the early learning curve. What sometimes comes as a wonderful surprise, though, is the intimacy breastfeeding adds to their relationship with their baby. Breastfeeding is far more than food. It is also a way of giving and receiving love.

Enjoy the early weeks and months with your baby! This is truly one of life's special times. And we promise—it really does get easier.

Resources

Throughout this book, we've described sources of help that might be of use to you. These additional resources will help you find specific items that you might need or in-person assistance.

Finding Local Sources of Help

The purpose of this section is to provide more information about some of the resources available to you locally and give you a starting point for finding these products and services.

Skilled Breastfeeding Help

Finding skilled help can be tricky, in part because there are different breastfeeding credentials reflecting different levels of education and training. Some of these initials, such as CLC, CLE, CBE, CBC, and LE, are awarded after attending a brief training course, usually no more than one week long. A person with these initials may be helpful but may have limited skills and understanding and limited experience working one on one with breastfeeding mothers and babies.

On the other hand, the credential IBCLC indicates a level of basic competency (at the very least) in the field of lactation. These initials stand for "international board-certified lactation consultant." To be awarded this credential, a person must pass an all-day certifying exam. But that is not all. To qualify to take that exam, she must first have a combination of formal education, breastfeeding education, and thousands of hours of working one on one with breastfeeding mothers and babies. The following are some ways you can find an IBCLC:

- Click on "Find a Lactation Consultant" on www.ilca.org. ILCA is the International Lactation Consultant Association, the professional association for lactation consultants. Not all international board-certified lactation consultants are members.

- Call your local hospital and ask to speak to the lactation consultant. Ask if she can help you or if she knows someone in your community who can.

- Check your telephone book under "Breastfeeding."

Another option is to contact a representative from a mother-to-mother breastfeeding group, such as La Leche League, Australian Breastfeeding Association, or Nursing Mothers Counsel. These women are volunteers who have breastfed their own children and have at least a basic understanding of breastfeeding. Some are highly skilled and some are relatively inexperienced. Ideally, if your problem is more complicated than they can help with, or if you need to be seen and they are unable to do so, they will refer you to someone in your area who can provide the help you need.

To find your local representative, go online:

- www.llli.org—La Leche League International

- www.breastfeeding.asn.au—Australian Breastfeeding Association

- www.nursingmothers.org—Nursing Mothers Counsel

Doulas

"Doula" comes from the Greek word for servant and refers to someone who provides practical and emotional help to women before, during, and after birth. To find local labor-support and postpartum doulas, contact www.dona.org—DONA International.

Breast Pumps, Rental or Purchase

To locate an Ameda rental pump or an Ameda Purely Yours personal pump near you, call Ameda Breastfeeding Products at 1-866-99AMEDA (1-866-992-6332), or go online to www.ameda.com.

To locate a Medela rental pump or a Medela Pump In Style purchase pump near you, contact Medela, Inc., at 1-800-TELLYOU (in the United States), or go online to www.medela.com.

An Accurate Baby Scale

The BabyWeigh scale by Medela is available for rent and is accurate to 0.1 oz., making it reliable enough to measure the milk a baby takes at the breast. (Medela's Baby Checker scale is not accurate enough for this purpose.)

To locate a BabyWeigh rental outlet near you, contact Medela at 1-800-TELLYOU (in the United States), or go online to www.medela.com.

To Prevent Milk Leakage

* www.lilypadz.com—Website for LilyPadz, the silicone product that prevents milk leakage

Websites of Interest

* www.breastfeedingmadesimple.com—Our website with lots of extras, including many additional links to relevant websites

* www.nancymohrbacher.com—Nancy's blog on breastfeeding research and trends and more

* www.uppitysciencechick.com—Kathy's website on the latest in breastfeeding, postpartum depression, mother-infant sleep, and health psychology

* www.infantrisk.org—The new website of Dr. Thomas Hale's Infant Risk Center provides information on the safety of

medications, over-the-counter products, and environmental contaminants. They can also be reached by telephone during business hours (U.S. central time) at 806-352-2519.

- www.bfmed.org/Resources/Protocols.aspx-—Academy of Breastfeeding Medicine's protocols on a variety of topics, ncluding co-sleeping and breastfeeding

- www.nd.edu/~jmckenn1/lab/—Website of James McKenna, researcher on parent-child co-sleeping

- http://bfar.org—Website of Diana West, IBCLC; for women who are breastfeeding after breast reduction surgery

- www.lowmilksupply.org—Website of Diana West and Lisa Marasco; for women who are concerned about their milk production

- www.biologicalnurturing.com—Website of British researcher Suzanne Colson, with information and video clips of laid-back breastfeeding

- www.postpartum.net—Keeps a listing of counselors who specialize in perinatal mental health (though, as with any health care provider, these counselors may or may not be knowledgeable about breastfeeding or supportive of your desire to continue)

Recommended Books and DVDs

The following books and DVDs by other authors are among our favorites. We also include two of our own.

Books and Articles

Hale, T. 2010. *Medications and Mothers' Milk*, 14th ed. Amarillo, TX: Hale Publishing. Available from www.ibreastfeeding.com.

Kendall-Tackett, K. A. 2005. *The Hidden Feelings of Motherhood*, 2nd ed. Amarillo, TX: Hale Publishing. Available from www.ibreast feeding.com.

Kendall-Tackett, K. A. 2009. Making peace with your birth experience. *New Beginnings* 5–6:50–55.

Mohrbacher, N. 2010. *Breastfeeding Answers Made Simple: A Guide for Helping Mothers*. Amarillo, TX: Hale Publishing. (For those who'd like to help other breastfeeding mothers.) Available from www. ibreastfeeding.com.

Palmer, G. 2009. *The Politics of Breastfeeding: Why Breasts Are Bad for Business*. London: Pinter & Martin.

Rapley, G., and T. Murkett. 2008. *Baby-Led Weaning: Helping Your Baby to Love Good Food*. London: Vermilion.

Simkin, P., and P. Klaus. 2004. *When Survivors Give Birth: Understanding and Healing the Effects of Early Sexual Abuse on Childbearing Women*. Seattle: Classic Day Publishing.

Smith, L. J. 2010. *Impact of Birthing Practices on Breastfeeding: Protecting the Mother and Baby Continuum*, 2nd ed. Boston: Jones and Bartlett.

Sperlich, M., and J. Seng. 2008. *Survivor Moms: Women's Stories of Birthing, Mothering and Health After Sexual Abuse*. Eugene, OR: Mother-baby Press.

Uvnäs-Moberg, K. 2003. *The Oxytocin Factor: Tapping the Hormone of Calm, Love and Healing*. New York: Da Capo Press.

West, D. 2001. *Defining Your Own Success: Breastfeeding After Breast Reduction Surgery*. Schaumburg, IL: La Leche League International.

West, D., and L. Marasco. 2009. *The Breastfeeding Mother's Guide to Making More Milk*. New York: McGraw-Hill.

DVDs

Bergman, N. 2000. *Kangaroo Mother Care: Restoring the Original Paradigm for Infant Care and Breastfeeding.* This video is available at www.geddesproduction.com and www.kangaroomothercare.com.

Colson, S. 2008. *Biological Nurturing: Laid-Back Breastfeeding.* Hythe, UK: The Nurturing Project. Available from www.biological nurturing.com and www.ibreastfeeding.com.

Smillie, C. 2007. *Baby-Led Breastfeeding: The Mother-Baby Dance.* Los Angeles: Geddes Production. Available from www.geddesproduction. com.

References

AAP (American Academy of Pediatrics, Committee on Drugs). 2001. The transfer of drugs and other chemicals into human milk. *Pediatrics* 108:776–789.

AAP (American Academy of Pediatrics, Subcommittee on Hyperbilirubinemia). 2004. Management of hyperbilirubinemia in the newborn infant 35 or more weeks of gestation. *Pediatrics* 114:297–316.

AAP (American Academy of Pediatrics, Task Force on Sudden Infant Death Syndrome). 2005a. The changing concept of Sudden Infant Death Syndrome: Diagnostic coding shifts, controversies regarding the sleeping environment, and new variables to consider in reducing risk. *Pediatrics* 116:1245–1255.

AAP (American Academy of Pediatrics, Work Group on Breastfeeding). 2005b. Breastfeeding and the use of human milk. *Pediatrics* 115:496–506.

Academy of Breastfeeding Medicine. 2008. Clinical protocol number 6: Guidelines on co-sleeping and breastfeeding. *Breastfeeding Medicine* 3:38–43. Available at www.bfmed.org.

Agostoni, C., T. Decsi, M. Fewtrell, O. Goulet, S. Kolacek, B. Koletzko, K. F. Michaelsen, L. Moreno, J. Puntis, J. Rigo, R. Shamir, H. Szajewska, D. Turck, J. van Goudoever, and ESPGHAN Committee on Nutrition. 2008. Complementary feeding: A commentary by the ESPGHAN Committee on Nutrition. *Journal of Pediatric Gastroenterology and Nutrition* 46(1):99–110.

Ainsworth, M. D. S., and J. Bowlby. 1991. An ethological approach to personality development. *American Psychologist* 46:333–341.

Anisfeld, E., V. Casper, M. Nozyce, and N. Cunningham. 1990. Does infant carrying promote attachment? An experimental study of the effects of increased physical contact on the development of attachment. *Child Development* 61:1617–1627.

APA (American Psychiatric Association). 2000. *Diagnostic and Statistical Manual of Mental Disorders*, 4th ed., text revision. Washington, DC: Author.

Armstrong, J., and J. Reilly. 2002. Breastfeeding and lowering the risk of childhood obesity. *Lancet* 359:2003–2004.

Ball, T. M., and A. L. Wright. 1999. Health care costs of formula-feeding in the first year of life. *Pediatrics* 103:870–876.

Bartick, M., and A. Reinhold. 2010. The burden of suboptimal breastfeeding in the United States: A pediatric cost analysis. *Pediatrics* 125(5):e1048–e1056.

Bates, J., C. Maslin, and K. Frankel. 1985. Attachment security, mother-child interaction, and temperament as predictors of behavior problem ratings at three years. In *Growing Points in Attachment Theory and Research. Monographs of the Society for Research in Child Development*, edited by I. Bretherton and E. Waters. Chicago: Society for Research in Child Development.

Benedict, M., L. Paine, and L. Paine. 1994. *Long-term Effects of Child Sexual Abuse on Functioning in Pregnancy and Pregnancy Outcome.* Final report, National Center on Child Abuse and Neglect. Washington, DC: National Center on Child Abuse and Neglect.

Benson, S. 2001. What is normal? A study of normal breastfeeding dyads during the first sixty hours of life. *Breastfeeding Review* 9:27–32.

Bergman, N. 2001a. Kangaroo Mother Care: Restoring the original paradigm for infant care and breastfeeding. Presentation at La Leche League International's 29th Annual Seminar for Physicians on Breastfeeding, Chicago, IL.

Bergman, N. 2001b. Kangaroo Mother Care: Restoring the original paradigm for infant care and breastfeeding. Video available at www.KangarooMotherCare.com.

Bergman, N., and N. Jurisoo. 1994. The "kangaroo-method" for treating low-birth-weight babies in a developing country. *Tropical Doctor* 24:57–60.

Bergman, N., L. Linley, and S. Fawcus. 2004. Randomized controlled trial of skin-to-skin contact from birth versus conventional incubator for physiological stabilization in 1200 to 2199 gram newborns. *Acta Paediatrica* 93:779–785.

Blumenthal, M., W. R. Busse, A. Goldberg, J. Gruenwald, T. Hall, S. Klein, C. W. Riggins, and R. S. Rister, eds. 1998. *The Complete German Commission E Monographs: Therapeutic Guide to Herbal Medicines.* Austin, TX: American Botanical Council.

Bramson, L., J. W. Lee, E. Moore, S. Montgomery, C. Neish, K. Bahjri, and C. L. Melcher. 2010. Effect of early skin-to-skin mother-infant contact during the first 3 hours following birth on exclusive breast-feeding during the maternity hospital stay. *Journal of Human Lactation* 26(2):130–137.

Brazelton, T. B., and J. K. Nugent. 1995. *Neonatal behavioral assessment scale.* London: MacKeith Press.

Bumgarner, N. J. 2000. *Mothering Your Nursing Toddler.* Schaumburg, IL: La Leche League International.

Bushnell, J., F. Sai, and J. Mullin. 1989. Neonatal recognition of the mother's face. *British Journal of Developmental Psychology* 7:3–15.

Cattaneo, A., R. Davanzo, B. Worku, A. Surjono, M. Echeverria, A. Bedri, E. Haksari, L. Osorno, B. Gudetta, D. Setyowireni, S. Quintero, and G. Tamburlini. 1998. Kangaroo Mother Care for low birthweight infants: A randomized control trial in different settings. *Acta Paediatrica* 87(9):976–985.

CDC (Centers for Disease Control and Prevention). 2010. *Breastfeeding Practices: Results from the 2006 National Immunization Survey.* www.cdc.gov/breastfeeding/data/NIS_data/index.htm. Accessed April 10, 2010.

Charpak, N., J. G. Ruiz-Peláez, C. Z. de Figueroa, and Y. Charpak. 2001. A randomized controlled trial of Kangaroo Mother Care: Results of follow-up at 1 year corrected age. *Pediatrics* 108(5):1072–1079.

Chen, A., and W. Rogan. 2004. Breastfeeding and the risk of postneo-natal death in the United States. *Pediatrics* 111:e435–e439.

Christensson K., T. Cabrera, E. Christensson, K. Uvnäs-Moberg, and J. Winberg. 1995. Separation distress call in the human neonate in the absence of maternal body contact. *Acta Paediatrica* 84(5):468–473.

Christensson, K., C. Siles, L. Moreno, A. Belaustequi, P. De La Fuente, H. Lagercrantz, P. Puyol, and J. Winberg. 1992. Temperature, metabolic adaptation and crying in healthy full-term newborns cared for skin to skin or in a cot. *Acta Paediatrica* 81(6–7):488–493.

Colson, S. 2005. Maternal breastfeeding positions: Have we got it right? (2). *Practising Midwife* 8(11):29–32.

Colson, S., L. DeRooy, and J. Hawdon. 2003. Biological Nurturing increases duration of breastfeeding for a vulnerable cohort. *MIDIRS Midwifery Digest* 13(1):92–97.

Colson, S. D., J. H. Meek, and J. M. Hawdon. 2008. Optimal positions for the release of primitive neonatal reflexes stimulating breastfeeding. *Early Human Development* 84:441–449.

Combs, V., and S. Marino. 1993. A comparison of growth patterns in breast and bottle-fed infants with congenital heart disease. *Pediatric Nursing* 19:175–179.

Coryllos, E., C. W. Genna, and A. C. Salloum. 2004. Congenital tongue-tie and its impact on breastfeeding. *Breastfeeding: Best for Baby and Mother.* American Academy of Pediatrics, Section on Breastfeeding newsletter (Summer):1–6.

Cregan, M., and P. Hartmann. 1999. Computerized breast measurement from conception to weaning: Clinical implications. *Journal of Human Lactation* 15:89–96.

Crockenberg, S., and K. McCluskey. 1986. Change in maternal behavior during the baby's first year of life. *Child Development* 57:746–753.

Cunha, M., J. Barreiros, I. Goncalves, and H. Figueiredo. 2009. Nutritive sucking pattern—from very low birth weight preterm to term newborn. *Early Human Development* 85:125–130.

Cunningham, A. S., D. B. Jelliffe, and E. F. Jelliffe. 1991. Breast-feeding and health in the 1980s: A global epidemiologic review. *Journal of Pediatrics* 118(5):659–666.

Daly, S. E., J. C. Kent, R. A. Owens, and P. E. Hartmann. 1996. Frequency and degree of milk removal and the short-term control of human milk synthesis. *Experimental Physiology* 81(5):861–875.

Daly, S., R. A. Owens, and P. E. Hartmann. 1993. The short-term synthesis and infant-regulated removal of milk in lactating women. *Experimental Physiology* 78(2):209–220.

de Carvalho, M., S. Robertson, A. Friedman, and M. Klaus. 1983. Effect of frequent breast feeding on early milk production and infant weight gain. *Pediatrics* 72:307–311.

de Carvalho, M., S. Robertson, and M. H. Klaus. 1984. Does the duration and frequency of early breastfeeding affect nipple pain? *Birth* 11(2):81–84.

DeMarzo, S., J. Seacat, and M. Neifert. 1991. Initial weight loss and return to birth weight criteria for breast-fed infants: Challenging the "rules of thumb." *American Journal of the Diseases of Children* 145:402.

Dennis, C. L., and K. McQueen. 2009. The relationship between infant-feeding outcomes and postpartum depression: A qualitative systematic review. *P ediatrics* 123(4):e736–e751.

Dettwyler, K. 1995. A time to wean: The hominid blueprint for the natural age of weaning in modern human populations. In *Breastfeeding: Biocultural Perspectives*, edited by P. Stuart-Macadam and K. Dettwyler. New York: Aldine de Gryter.

Doan, T., A. Gardiner, C. L. Gay, and K. A. Lee. 2007. Breast-feeding increases sleep duration of new parents. *Journal of Perinatal and Neonatal Nursing* 21(3):200–206.

Dodd, V., and C. Chalmers. 2003. Comparing the use of hydrogel dressings to lanolin ointment with lactating mothers. *Journal of Obstetric, Gynecologic, and Neonatal Nursing* 32:486–494.

Dorheim, S. K., G. T. Bondevik, M. Eberhard-Gran, and B. Bjorvatn. 2009. Sleep and depression in postpartum women: A population-based study. *Sleep* 32(7):847–855.

Duncan, B., J. Ey, C. J. Holberg, A. L. Wright, F. D. Martinez, and L. M. Taussig. 1993. Exclusive breast-feeding for at least 4 months protects against otitis media. *Pediatrics* 91(5):867–872.

Dunham, C. 1992. *Mamatoto: A Celebration of Birth.* New York: Viking Penguin.

Dusdieker, L., B. M. Booth, P. J. Stumbo, and J. M Eichenberger. 1985. Effect of supplemental fluids on human milk production. *Journal of Pediatrics* 106(2):207–211.

Eisenberg, A., H. Murkoff, and S. Hathaway. 1989. *What to Expect the First Year.* New York: Workman Publishing Company.

Feldman, R., M. Keren, O. Gross-Rozval, and S. Tyano. 2004. Mother-child touch patterns in infant feeding disorders: Relation to maternal, child, and environmental factors. *Journal of the American Academy of Child and Adolescent Psychiatry* 43(9):1089–1097.

Feldman, R., A. Weller, J. F. Leckman, J. Kuint, and A. I. Eidelman. 1999. The nature of the mother's tie to her infant: Maternal bonding under conditions of proximity, separation, and potential loss. *Journal of Child Psychology and Psychiatry* 40:929–939.

Feldman, R., A. Weller, L. Sirota, and A. I. Eidelman. 2002. Skin-to-skin contact (Kangaroo Care) promotes self-regulation in premature infants: Sleep-wake cyclicity, arousal modulation, and sustained exploration. *Developmental Psychology* 38(2):194–197.

Fifer, W., and C. Moon. 1994. The role of the mother's voice in the organization of brain function in the newborn. *Acta Paediatrica Supplementum* 397:86–93.

Freed, G. L., S. J. Clark, J. A. Lohr, and J. R. Sorenson. 1995. Pediatrician involvement in breastfeeding promotion: A national study of residents and practitioners. *Pediatrics* 96:490–494.

Freed, G. L., S. J. Clark, J. R. Sorenson, J. A. Lohr, R. Cefalo, and P. Curtis. 1995. National assessment of physicians' breastfeeding knowledge, attitudes, training, and experience. *Journal of the American Medical Association* 273:472–476.

Freeman, M. P., J. R. Hibbeln, K. L. Wisner, J. M. Davis, D. Mischoulon, M. Peet, P. E. Keck Jr., L. B. Marangell, A. J. Richardson, J. Lake, and A. L. Stoll. 2006. Omega-3 fatty acids: Evidence basis for treatment and future research in psychiatry. *Journal of Clinical Psychiatry* 67:1954–1967.

Gay, C. L., K. A. Lee, and S. Y. Lee. 2004. Sleep patterns and fatigue in new mothers and fathers. *Biological Research for Nursing* 5(4):311–318.

Glover, R., and D. Wiessinger. 2008. The infant-mother breastfeeding conversation: Helping when they lose the thread. In *Supporting Sucking Skills in Breastfeeding Infants*, edited by Catherine Watson Genna. Boston: Jones and Bartlett.

Goldman, A., A. S. Garza, and R. M. Goldblum. 1983. Immunologic components in human milk during the second year of lactation. *Acta Paediatrica Scandinavia* 72:461–462.

Grajeda, R., and R. Perez-Escamilla. 2002. Stress during labor and delivery is associated with delayed onset of lactation among urban Guatemalan women. *Journal of Nutrition* 132:3055–3060.

Greer, F. R., S. H. Sicherer, and A. W. Burks. 2008. Effects of early nutritional interventions on the development of atopic disease in infants and children: the role of maternal dietary restriction, breastfeeding, timing of introduction of complementary foods, and hydrolyzed formulas. *Pediatrics* 121(1):183–191.

Groer, M. W., and M. W. Davis. 2006. Cytokines, infections, stress, and dysphoric moods in breastfeeders and formula feeders. *Journal of Obstetric, Gynecologic, and Neonatal Nursing* 35(5):599–607.

Groer, M. W., M. W. Davis, and J. Hemphill. 2002. Postpartum stress: Current concepts and the possible protective role of breastfeeding. *Journal of Obstetric, Gynecologic, and Neonatal Nursing* 31(4):411–417.

Gulick, E. 1986. The effects of breastfeeding on toddler health. *Pediatric Nursing* 12:51–54.

Hale, T. 2010. *Medications and Mothers' Milk*, 14th ed. Amarillo, TX: Hale Publishing.

Hammond, K. A. 1997. Adaptation of the maternal intestine during lactation. *Journal of Mammary Gland Biology and Neoplasia* 2:243–252.

Harlow, H. F. 1959. The nature of love. *American Psychologist* 13:573–685.

Hanson, L. 2004. *Immunobiology of Human Milk: How Human Milk Protects Infants.* Amarillo, TX: Pharmasoft Publishing.

Hausman, B. 2003. A formal look at formula promotion. Presentation at the International Lactation Consultant Association, Sydney, Australia.

Heinrichs, M., G. Meinlschmidt, I. Neumann, S. Wagner, C. Kirschbaum, U. Ehlert, and D. Hellhammer. 2001. Effects of suckling on hypothalamic-pituitary-adrenal axis responses to psychosocial stress in postpartum lactating women. *Journal of Clinical Endocrinology & Metabolism* 86(10):4798–4804.

Heinrichs, M., I. Neumann, and U. Ehlert. 2002. Lactation and stress: Protective effects of breast-feeding in humans. *Stress* 5(3):195–203.

Helm, A. 2004. Post on Lactnet, lactation professional listserv, August 15, 2004. Reprinted with permission.

Hibbeln, J. R. 2002. Seafood consumption, the DHA content of mothers' milk and prevalence rates of postpartum depression: A cross-national, ecological analysis. *Journal of Affective Disorders* 69:15–29.

Hill, P. D., Aldag, J. C., Zinaman, M., and R. T. Chatterton Jr. 2007. Comparison of milk output between breasts in pump-dependent mothers. *Journal of Human Lactation* 23:333–337.

Hillervik-Lindquist, C., Y. Hofvander, and S. Sjölin. 1991. Studies on perceived breast milk insufficiency: III. Consequences for breast milk consumption and growth. *Acta Paediatrica Scandinavia* 80(3):297–303.

Holliday, K. E., J. R. Allen, D. L. Waters, M. A. Gruca, S. M. Thompson, and K. J. Gaskin. 1991. Growth of human milk-fed and formula-fed infants with cystic fibrosis. *Journal of Pediatrics* 118(1):77–79.

Høst, A. 1991. Importance of the first meal on the development of cow's milk allergy and intolerance. *Allergy Proceedings* 12:227–232.

Humphrey, S. 2003. *The Nursing Mother's Herbal.* Minneapolis: Fairview Press.

Hurst, N. M., C. J. Valentine, L. Renfro, P. Burns, and L. Ferlic. 1997. Skin-to-skin holding in the neonatal intensive care unit influences maternal milk volume. *Journal of Perinatology* 17(3):213–217.

ILCA (International Lactation Consultant Association). 2005. *Clinical Guidelines for the Establishment of Exclusive Breastfeeding.* Raleigh, NC: International Lactation Consultant Association.

Illingsworth, P. J., R. T. Jung, P. W. Howie, P. Leslie, and T. E. Isles. 1986. Diminution in energy expenditure during lactation. *British Medical Journal* (Clinical Research edition) 292(6518):437–441.

Ip, S., M. Chung, G. Raman, P. Chew, N. Magula, D. DeVine, T. Trikalinos, and J. Lau. 2007. Breastfeeding and maternal and infant health outcomes in developed countries. Evidence Report—Technology Assessment (Full Report) 153:1–186.

Ip, S., M. Chung, G. Raman, T. A. Trikalinos, and J. Lau. 2009. A summary of the Agency for Healthcare Research and Quality's evidence report on breastfeeding in developed countries. *Breastfeeding Medicine* 4:S17–S30.

Jacobs, L. A., J. E. Dickinson, P. D. Hart, D. A. Doherty, and S. J. Faulkner. 2007. Normal nipple position in term infants measured on breastfeeding ultrasound. *Journal of Human Lactation* 23:52–59.

Johnston, C. C., B. Stevens, J. Pinelli, S. Gibbins, F. Filion, A. Jack, S. Steele, K. Boyer, and A. Veilleux. 2003. Kangaroo Care is effective in diminishing pain response in preterm neonates. *Archives of Pediatric and Adolescent Medicine* 157:1084–1088.

Jones, G.,R. W. Steketee, R. E. Black, Z. A. Bhutta, S. S. Morris, and Bellagio Child Survival Study Group. 2003. How many child deaths can we prevent this year? *Lancet* 362(9377):65–71.

Jones, N. A., B. A. McFall, and M. A. Diego. 2004. Patterns of brain electical activity in infants of depressed mothers who breast-feed and bottle-feed: The mediating role of infant temperament. *Biological Psychology* 67:103–124.

Kashaninia, Z., F. Sajedi, M. Rahgozar, and F. A. Noghabi. 2008. The effect of Kangaroo Care on behavioral responses to pain of an intramuscular injection in neonates. *Journal for Specialists in Pediatric Nursing* 13(4):275–280.

Keane, V., et al. 1988. Do solids help baby sleep through the night? *American Journal of Diseases of Childhood* 142:404–405.

Kearney, M., and L. Cronenwett. 1991. Breastfeeding and employment. *Journal of Obstetric, Gynecologic, and Neonatal Nursing* 20:471–480.

Kendall-Tackett, K. A. 2004. *Breastfeeding and the Sexual Abuse Survivor.* Lactation Consultant Series 2, Unit 9. Schaumburg, IL: La Leche League International.

Kendall-Tackett, K. A. 2008. *Clinics in Human Lactation: Non-pharmacologic treatments for depression in new mothers: Evidence-Based Support of Omega-3s, Bright Light Therapy, Exercise, Social Support, Psychotherapy and St. John's Wort.* Amarillo, TX: Hale Publishing.

Kendall-Tackett, K. A. 2010a. *Depression in New Mothers: Causes, Consequences, and Treatment* Options, 2nd ed. London: Routledge.

Kendall-Tackett, K. A. Forthcoming. Omega-3 fatty acids and women's mental health in the perinatal period. *Journal of Midwifery & Women's Health.*

Kendall-Tackett, K. A., ed. 2010b. *The Psychoneuroimmunology of Chronic Disease: Exploring the Links Between Inflammation, Stress, and Illness.* Washington, DC: American Psychological Association.

Kendall-Tackett, K. A., and T. W. Hale. 2010c. Use of antidepressants in pregnant and breastfeeding women: A review and synthesis of recent studies. *Journal of Human Lactation* 26(2):187–195.

Kendall-Tackett, K. A., and M. Sugarman. 1995. The social consequences of long-term breastfeeding. *Journal of Human Lactation* 11:179–183.

Kent, J. C. 2007. How breastfeeding works. *Journal of Midwifery & Women's Health* 52:564–570.

Kent, J. C., L. R. Mitoulas, M. Cregan, D. Ramsay, D. A. Doherty, and P. E. Hartmann. 2006. Volume and frequency of breastfeedings and fat content of breast milk throughout the day. *Pediatrics* 117:e387–e395.

Kirsten, G. F., N. J. Bergman, and F. M. Hann. 2001. Kangaroo mother care in the nursery. *Pediatric Clinics of North America* 48(2):443–452.

Klaus, M. H., J. H. Kennell, and P. H. Klaus. 1996. *Bonding: Building the Foundations of Secure Attachment and Independence.* New York: Da Capo Press.

Klaus, M., and P. Klaus. 2000. *Your Amazing Newborn.* New York: Perseus Books.

Konner, M. 1976. Maternal care, infant behavior and development among the !Kung. In *Kalahari Hunter-gatherers: Studies of the !Kung San and Their Neighbors,* edited by R. B. Lee and I. DeVore. Cambridge, MA: Harvard University Press.

Kramer, M. S., F. Aboud, E. Mironova, I. Vanilovich, R. W. Platt, L. Matush, et al. 2008. Breastfeeding and child cognitive development: New evidence from a large randomized trial. *Archives of General Psychiatry* 65(5):578–584.

Kramer, M. S., T. Guo, R. W. Platt, I. Vanilovich, Z. Sevkovskaya, L. Dzikovich, K. F. Michaelson, K. Dewey, and Promotion of Breastfeeding Intervention Trials Study Group. 2004. Feeding effects on growth during infancy. *Journal of Pediatrics* 145(5):600–605.

Labbok, M. H., D. Clark, and A. S. Goldman. 2004. Breastfeeding: Maintaining an irreplaceable immunological resource. *Nature Reviews/Immunology* 4:565–572.

Lawrence, R., and R. Lawrence. 2005. *Breastfeeding: A Guide for the Medical Profession.* St. Louis, MO: Elsevier Mosby.

Lewis, T., F. Amini, and R. Lannon. 2000. *A General Theory of Love.* New York: Vintage.

Li, R., S. B. Fein, and L. M. Grummer-Strawn. 2008. Association of breastfeeding intensity and bottle-emptying behaviors at early infancy with infants' risk for excess weight at late infancy. *Pediatrics* 122(Supplement 2):S77–S84.

Ludington-Hoe, S. M., with S. K. Golant. 1993. *Kangaroo Care: The Best You Can Do to Help Your Preterm Infant.* New York: Bantam.

Macknin, M., S. V. Medendorp, and M. C. Maier. 1989. Infant sleep and bedtime cereal. *American Journal of the Diseases of Childhood* 143(9):1066–1068.

Matthieson, A., A. Ransjö-Arvidson, E. Nissen, and K. Uvnäs-Moberg. 2001. Postpartum maternal oxytocin release by newborns: Effects of infant hand massage and sucking. *Birth* 28:13–19.

McCarter-Spaulding, D., and J. A. Horowitz. 2007. How does postpartum depression affect breastfeeding? *American Journal of Maternal/ Child Nursing* 32(1):10–17.

McNamara, R. K. 2009. Evaluation of docosahexaenoic acid deficiency as a preventable risk factor for recurrent affective disorders: Current status, future directions, and dietary recommendations. *Prostaglandins, Leukotrienes, and Essential Fatty Acids* 81:223–231.

Mead, M., and N. Newton. 1967. Cultural patterns of perinatal behavior. In *Childbearing: Its Social and Psychological Aspects*, edited by S. Richardson and A. Guttmacher. Baltimore: Williams & Wilkins.

Mezzacappa, E. S., and E. S. Katkin. 2002. Breastfeeding is associated with reduced perceived stress and negative mood in mothers. *Health Psychology* 21:187–193.

Michelsson K., K. Christensson, H. Rothgänger, and J. Winberg. 1996. Crying in separated and non-separated newborns: Sound spectrographic analysis. *Acta Paediatrica* 85(4):471–475.

Mikiel-Kostyra, K., J. Mazur, and I. Boltruszko. 2002. Effect of early skin to skin contact after delivery on duration of breastfeeding: A prospective cohort study. *Acta Paediatrica* 91:1301–1367.

Milligan, R. A., P. M. Flenniken, and L. C. Pugh. 1996. Positioning intervention to minimize fatigue in breastfeeding women. *Applied Nursing Research* 9(2):67–70.

Mitoulas, L., C. T. Lai, L. C. Gurrin, M. Larsson, and P. E. Hartmann. 2002. Efficacy of breast milk expression using an electric breast pump. *Journal of Human Lactation* 18(4):344–351.

Mohrbacher, N. 1993. How often should a baby breastfeed? *BabyTalk* (September):40–41.

Mohrbacher, N. 1995. *Approaches to Weaning*. Publication no. 307–17. Schaumburg, IL: La Leche League International.

Mohrbacher, N. 2010. *Breastfeeding Answers Made Simple: A Guide for Helping Mothers*. Amarillo, TX: Hale Publishing.

Molbak, K., A. Gottschau, P. Aaby, N. Hojlyng, L. Ingholt, and A. P. J. Da Silva. 1994. Prolonged breast feeding, diarrhoeal disease, and survival of children in Guinea-Bissau. *British Medical Journal* 308:1403–1406.

Montagu, A. 1978. *Touching: The Human Significance of the Skin.* New York: Harper & Row.

Mooncey, S. 1997. The effect of mother-infant skin-to-skin contact on plasma cortisol and beta-endorphin concentrations in preterm newborns. *Infant Behavior and Development* 20:553.

Moore, E. R., G. C. Anderson, and N. J. Bergman. 2007. Early skin-to-skin contact for mothers and their healthy newborn infants. *Cochrane Database of Systematic Reviews,* 3(10.1022/14651858. CD003519.pub2).

Motil, K. J., H. P. Sheng, C. M. Montandon, and W. W. Wong. 1997. Human milk protein does not limit growth of breast-fed infants. *Journal of Pediatric Gastroenterology and Nutrition* 24(1):10–17.

Nehlig, A., and G. Debry. 1994. Consequences on the newborn of chronic maternal coffee during gestation and lactation: A review. *Journal of the American College of Nutrition* 13:6–21.

Neville, M. C., R. Keller, J. Seacat, V. Lutes, M. Neifert, C. Casey, J. Allen, and P. Archer. 1988. Studies in human lactation: Milk volumes in lactating women during the onset of lactation and full lactation. *American Journal of Clinical Nutrition* 48(6):1375–1386.

Newman, J., and T. Pitman. 2006. *The Ultimate Breastfeeding Book of Answers.* New York, NY: Three Rivers Press.

Newton, N. 1978. The role of oxytocin reflexes in three interpersonal reproductive acts: Coitus, birth, and breastfeeding. *Clinical Psychoneuroendocrinology in Reproduction* 22:411–418.

Noel-Weiss, J., G. Courant, and A. K. Woodend. 2008. Physiological weight loss in the breastfed neonate: A systematic review. *Open Medicine* 2:E11–E22.

Nommsen-Rivers, L. A., M. J. Heinig, R. J. Cohen, and K. G. Dewey. 2008. Newborn wet and soiled diaper counts and timing of onset of lactation as indicators of breastfeeding inadequacy. *Journal of Human Lactation* 24:27–33.

Novello, A. 1990. You can eat healthy. *Parade* (November 11):5.

Nyqvist, K. H. 2008. Early attainment of breastfeeding competence in very preterm infants. *Acta Paediatrica* 97:776–781.

Parmar, V. R., A. Kumar, R. Kaur, S. Parmar, D. Kaur, S. Basu, S. Jain, and S. Narula. 2009. Experience with Kangaroo mother care in a neonatal intensive care unit (NICU) in Chandigarh, India. *Indian Journal of Pediatrics* 76(1):25–28.

PDR Staff. 2010 *Physicians' Desk Reference*. New York: PDR Network, LLC.

Polan, H. J., and M. Ward. 1994. Role of the mother's touch in failure to thrive: A preliminary investigation. *Journal of the American Academy of Child and Adolescent Psychiatry* 33:1098–1105.

Prentice, A. 1989. Evidence for local feedback control of human milk secretion. *Biochemical Society Transactions* 17:489–492.

Prentice, A. M., S. B. Roberts, A. Prentice, A. A. Paul, M. Watkinson, A. A. Watkinson, and R. G. Whitehead. 1983. Dietary supplementation of lactating Gambian women. I. Effect on breast-milk volume and quality. *Human Nutrition: Clinical Nutrition* 37(1):53–64.

Prentice, J. C., M. C. Lu, L. Lange, and N. Halfon. 2002. The association between reported childhood sexual abuse and breastfeeding initiation. *Journal of Human Lactation* 18:219–226.

Quillin, S., and L. L. Glenn. 2004. Interaction between feeding method and co-sleeping on maternal-newborn sleep. *Journal of Obstetric, Gynecologic, and Neonatal Nursing* 33:580–588.

Ram, K. T., P. Bobby, S. M. Hailpern, J. C. Lo, M. Schocken, J. Skurnick, and N. Santoro. 2008. Duration of lactation is associated with lower prevalence of the metabolic syndrome in midlife—SWAN, the study of women's health across the nation. *American Journal of Obstetrics and Gynecology* 198:e261–e266.

Ramsay, D. T., J. C. Kent, R. A. Owens, and P. E. Hartmann. 2004. Ultrasound imaging of milk ejection in the breast of lactating women. *Pediatrics* 113(2):361–367.

Ransjö-Arvidson, A.-B., A.-S. Matthiesen, G. Lilja, E. Nissen, A.-M. Widström, and K. Uvnäs-Moberg. 2001. Maternal analgesia during labor disturbs newborn behavior: Effects on breastfeeding, temperature, and crying. *Birth* 28:5–12.

Rapley, G., and T. Murkett. 2008. *Baby-led Weaning: Helping Your Baby to Love Good Food.* London: Ebury Publishing.

Rees, A.-M., M.-P. Austin, and G. Parker. 2005. Role of omega-3 fatty acids as a treatment for depression in the perinatal period. *Australia & New Zealand Journal of Psychiatry* 39:274–280.

Righard, L. 1998. Are breastfeeding problems related to incorrect breastfeeding technique and the use of pacifiers and bottles? *Birth* 25:40–44.

Righard, L., and M. Alade. 1990. Effect of delivery room routines on success of first breast feed. *Lancet* 336(8723):1105–1107.

Riva, E., C. Agostoni, G. Biasucci, S. Trojan, D. Luotti, L. Fiori, and M. Giovannini. 1996. Early breastfeeding is linked to higher intelligence quotient scores in dietary treated phenylketonuric children. *Acta Paediatrica* 85(1):56–58.

Roche-Paull, R. 2010 *Breastfeeding in Combat Boots.* Amarillo, TX: Hale Publishing.

Rogers, C. S., S. Morris, and L. J. Taper. 1987. Weaning from the breast: Influences on maternal decisions. *Pediatric Nursing* 13:341–345.

Rosin, H. 2009. The case against breastfeeding. *Atlantic* (April) www.theatlantic.com/magazine/archive/2009/04/the-case-against-breast-feeding/7311/1/. Accessed April 4, 2010.

Rowe-Murray, H. J., and J. R. W. Fisher. 2002. Baby friendly hospital practices: Cesarean section is a persistent barrier to early initiation of breastfeeding. *Birth* 29:124–131.

Sacker, A., M. A. Quigley, and Y. J. Kelly. 2006. Breastfeeding and developmental delay: Findings from the millennium cohort study. *Pediatrics* 118:e682–e689.

Schulte, P. 1995. Minimizing alcohol exposure of the breastfeeding infant. *Journal of Human Lactation* 11:317–319.

Schwarz, E. B., R. M. Ray, A. M. Stuebe, M. A. Allison, R. B. Ness, M. S. Freiberg, and J. A. Cauley. 2009. Duration of lactation and risk factors for maternal cardiovascular disease. *Obstetrics and Gynecology* 113(5):974–982.

Seammon, R. E., and L. Q. Doyle. 1920. Observations on the capacity of the stomach in the first ten days of postnatal life. *American Journal of the Diseases of Children* 20:516–538.

Sepkoski, C. M., B. M. Lester, G. W. Ostheimer, and T. B. Brazelton. 1992. The effects of maternal epidural anesthesia on neonatal behavior during the first month. *Developmental Medicine and Child Neurology* 34(12):1072–1080.

Shah, V., A. Taddio, and M. J. Rieder. 2009. Effectiveness and tolerability of pharmacologic and combined interventions for reducing injection pain during routine childhood immunizations: Systematic review and meta-analyses. *Clinical Therapeutics* 31:S104–S151.

Shaw, R. J., T. Deblois, L. Ikuta, K. Ginzburg, B. Fleisher, and C. Koopman. 2006. Acute stress disorder among parents of infants in the neonatal intensive care nursery. *Psychosomatics* 47(3):206–212.

Shonkoff, J. P., W. T. Boyce, and B. S. McEwen. 2009. Neuroscience, molecular biology, and the childhood roots of health disparities: Building a new framework for health promotion and disease prevention. *Journal of the American Medical Association* 301(21):2252–2259.

Shrago, L. C., E. Reifsnider, and K. Insel. 2006. The neonatal bowel output study: Indicators of adequate breast milk intake in neonates. *Pediatric Nursing* 32:195–201.

Small, M. F. 1998. *Our Babies, Ourselves: How Biology and Culture Shape the Way We Parent.* New York: Anchor.

Smillie, C. 2008. How infants learn to feed: A neurobehavioral model. In *Supporting Sucking Skills in Breastfeeding Infants*, edited by C. W. Genna. Boston: Jones and Bartlett.

Smith, L. J. 2010. *Impact of Birthing Practices on Breastfeeding.* Boston: Jones and Bartlett.

Stern, G., and L. Kruckman. 1983. Multi-disciplinary perspectives on postpartum depression: An anthropological critique. *Social Science and Medicine* 17:1027–1041.

Stettler, N., V. A. Stallings, A. B. Troxel, J. Zhao, R. Schinnar, S. E. Nelson, E. E. Ziegler, and B. L. Strom. 2005. Weight gain in the first week of life and overweight in adulthood: A cohort study of European American subjects fed infant formula. *Circulation* 111:1897–1903.

Su, D., Y. Zhao, C. Binna, J. Scott, and W. Oddy. 2007. Breast-feeding mothers can exercise: Results of a cohort study. *Public Health Nutrition* 10:1089–1093.

Sugarman, M., and K. A. Kendall-Tackett. 1995. Weaning ages in a sample of American women who practice extended breastfeeding. *Clinical Pediatrics* 34:642–647.

Tappin, D., R. Ecob, S. Stat, and H. Brooke. 2005. Bedsharing, room-sharing, and sudden infant death syndrome in Scotland: A case-control study. *Journal of Pediatrics* 147:32–37.

Taveras, E. M., A. M. Capra, P. A. Braveman, N. G. Jensvold, G. J. Escobar, and T. Lieu, 2003. Clinician support and psychosocial risk factors associated with breastfeeding discontinuation. *Pediatrics* 112:108–115.

Törnhage, C.-J., E. Stuge, T. Lindberg, and F. Serenius. 1999. First week Kangaroo Care in sick, very preterm infants. *Acta Paediatrica* 88(12):1402–1404.

Toschke, A. M., J. Vignerova, L. Lhotska, K. Osancova, B. Koletzko, and R. von Kries. 2002. Overweight and obesity in 6- to 14-year-old Czech children in 1991: Protective effect of breast-feeding. *Journal of Pediatrics* 141(6):764–769.

Uvnäs-Moberg, K. 1998. Oxytocin may mediate the benefits of positive social interaction and emotions. *Psychoneuroendocrinology* 23:819–835.

Uvnäs-Moberg, K. 2003. *The oxytocin factor: Tapping the hormone of calm, love, and healing.* Cambridge, MA: Da Capo Press.

Uvnäs-Moberg, K., A. M. Widström, G. Marchinin, and J. Winberg. 1987. Release of GI hormones in mothers and infants by sensory stimulation. *Acta Paediatrica Scandanavia* 76(6):851–860.

Wagner, C. L., with S. N. Taylor and B. W. Hollis. 2010. *New Insights into Vitamin D During Pregnancy, Lactation and Early Infancy.* Amarillo, TX: Hale Publishing.

Wallace, J. P., G. Inbar, and K. Ernsthausen. 1992. Infant acceptance of postexercise breast milk. *Pediatrics* 89(6, pt.2):1245–1247.

Watson, J. B. 1928. *Psychological Care of the Infant and Child.* New York: W. W. Norton & Co.

WebMD. 2010. Breastfeeding hints and hurdles. www.webmd.com /parenting/baby/breastfeeding-9/slideshow-breastfeeding. Accessed January 30, 2010.

West, D. 2001. *Defining Your Own Success: Breastfeeding After Breast Reduction Surgery.* Schaumburg, IL: La Leche League International.

WHO (World Health Organization). 2001. *The Optimal Duration of Exclusive Breastfeeding: Report of an Expert Consultation.* Geneva: World Health Organization.

WHO (World Health Organization). 2006. Breastfeeding in the WHO Multicentre Growth Reference Study. *Acta Paediatrica Supplement* 450:16–26.

WHO (World Health Organization). 2009. *Infant and young child feeding: Model chapter for textbooks for medical students and allied health professionals.* Geneva: World Health Organization.

Wiessinger, D. 1998. A breastfeeding tool using a sandwich analogy for latch-on. *Journal of Human Lactation* 14:51–56.

Willis, C., and V. Livingstone. 1995. Infant insufficient milk syndrome associated with maternal postpartum hemorrhage. *Journal of Human Lactation* 11:123–126.

Woodbury, R. M. 1925. *Infant Mortality and Its Causes.* Baltimore: Williams & Wilkins.

Woolridge, M., and C. Fisher. 1988. Colic, "overfeeding," and symptoms of lactose malabsorption in the breast-fed baby: A possible artifact of feed management? *Lancet* 2(8605):382–384.

Yamauchi, Y., and I. Yamanouchi. 1990. Breast-feeding frequency during the first 24 hours after birth in full-term neonates. *Pediatrics* 82:171–175.

Zangen, S., C. Di Lorenzo, T. Zangen, H. Mertz, L. Schwankovsky, and P. E. Hyman. 2001. Rapid maturation of gastric relaxation in newborn infants. *Pediatric Research* 50(5):629–632.

Nancy Mohrbacher, IBCLC, FILCA, is an international board-certified lactation consultant based in the Chicago, IL, area, who breastfed her three sons and has worked one-on-one with thousands of breastfeeding families since 1982. Her books on breastfeeding are widely used by both professionals and parents. In 2008, she was in the first group of sixteen lactation consultants whose lifetime achievements in breastfeeding were recognized with the designation Fellow of the International Lactation Consultant Association. She is a popular speaker at breastfeeding conferences for parents and professionals around the world.

Kathleen Kendall-Tackett, Ph.D., IBCLC, is a health psychologist and international board-certified lactation consultant based in Amarillo, TX, who breastfed her two sons and has been working with breastfeeding families since 1994. She is clinical associate professor of pediatrics at Texas Tech University School of Medicine, has authored or edited twenty books and is editor of the journal *Clinical Lactation*. She is a popular speaker at conferences for parents and professionals around the world.

Foreword writer **Jack Newman, MD,** is a pediatrician and author of *The Ultimate Breastfeeding Book of Answers*. He is a graduate of the University of Toronto medical school. He started the first hospital-based breastfeeding clinic in Canada in 1984 and has consulted with UNICEF for the Baby Friendly Hospital Initiative in Africa. Newman has practiced as a physician in Canada, New Zealand, and South Africa.

Index

MORE BOOKS *from*
NEW HARBINGER PUBLICATIONS

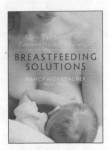

**BREASTFEEDING
SOLUTIONS**

Quick Tips for the Most
Common Nursing Challenges

978-1608825578 / US $15.95

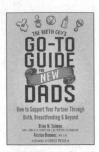

**THE BIRTH GUY'S GO-TO
GUIDE FOR NEW DADS**

How to Support Your
Partner Through Birth,
Breastfeeding & Beyond

978-1684031597 / US $16.95

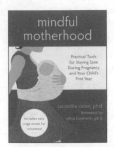

MINDFUL MOTHERHOOD

Practical Tools for Staying
Sane During Pregnancy &
Your Child's First Year

978-1572246294 / US $17.95

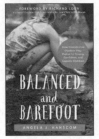

BALANCED & BAREFOOT

How Unrestricted Outdoor
Play Makes for Strong,
Confident & Capable Children

978-1626253735 / US $16.95

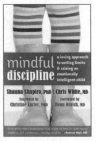

MINDFUL DISCIPLINE

A Loving Approach to
Setting Limits & Raising an
Emotionally Intelligent Child

978-1608828845 / US $17.95

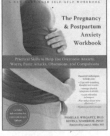

**THE PREGNANCY &
POSTPARTUM ANXIETY
WORKBOOK**

Practical Skills to Help You
Overcome Anxiety,
Worry, Panic Attacks,
Obsessions & Compulsions

978-1572245891 / US $23.95

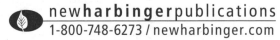

newharbingerpublications
1-800-748-6273 / newharbinger.com

(VISA, MC, AMEX / prices subject to change without notice)

Follow Us

Don't miss out on new books in the subjects that interest you.
Sign up for our Book Alerts at **newharbinger.com/bookalerts**